MASTERING IRIS REPAIR

A Video Textbook of Iris Repair and Pupilloplasty Techniques

MASTERING IRIS REPAIR

A Video Textbook of Iris Repair and Pupilloplasty Techniques

Editors

Ashvin Agarwal, MBBS, MS
Chief of Clinical Services
Director
Dr. Agarwal's Group of Eye Hospitals and
Eye Research Centre
Chennai, India

Amar Agarwal, MS, FRCS, FRCOphth
Chairman and Managing Director
Dr. Agarwal's Group of Eye Hospitals and
Eye Research Centre
Chennai, India

Associate Editor
Priya Narang, MS
Director
Narang Eye Care & Laser Centre
Ahmedabad, India

CRC Press
Taylor & Francis Group
Boca Raton London New York

CRC Press is an imprint of the
Taylor & Francis Group an **informa** business

First published 2021 by SLACK Incorporated

Published 2024 by CRC Press
2385 NW Executive Center Drive, Suite 320, Boca Raton FL 33431

and by CRC Press
4 Park Square, Milton Park, Abingdon, Oxon, OX14 4RN

CRC Press is an imprint of Taylor & Francis Group, LLC

Cover Artist: Katherine Christie

Library of Congress Cataloging-in-Publication Data
Names: Agarwal, Ashvin, editor. | Agarwal, Amar, editor. | Narang, Priya, editor.
Title: Mastering iris repair : a video textbook of iris repair and pupilloplasty techniques / editors, Ashvin Agarwal, Amar Agarwal ; associate editor, Priya Narang.
Description: Thorofare, NJ : SLACK Incorporated, [2021] | Includes bibliographical references and index.
Identifiers: LCCN 2020018755 (print) | ISBN 9781630917265 (paperback) | ISBN 9781630917289
Subjects: MESH: Iris Diseases--surgery | Iris--surgery | Pupil Disorders--surgery | Reconstructive Surgical Procedures--methods
Classification: LCC RE352 (print) | NLM WW 240 | DDC 617.7/2--dc23
LC record available at https://lccn.loc.gov/2020018755

ISBN: 9781630917265 (pbk)
ISBN: 9781003525028 (ebk)

DOI: 10.1201/9781003525028

Additional resources can be found at
https://www.routledge.com/9781630917265

Dedication

This book is dedicated to George O. Waring IV, MD, FACS, a great human being and surgeon.

Contents

Website Contents

ACKNOWLEDGMENT

Nothing in this world moves without HIM and so also this book was only written by HIM.

About the Editors

Ashvin Agarwal, MBBS, MS is Chief of Clinical Services and Director of Dr. Agarwal's Group of Eye Hospitals and Eye Research Centre, which has more than 97 hospitals worldwide, and a subcommittee member of the International Society of Refractive Surgery. He is a cataract, cornea, and refractive surgeon with a special interest in handling complex and complicated cases, such as nucleus drop, IOL drop, trauma, iris and anterior segment reconstruction, and corneal decompensation. Dr. Agarwal was instrumental in performing a new form of surgery called *vitrectomy-assisted phacoemulsification* for aqueous misdirection syndrome. He also started the extrusion cannula-assisted levitation technique for dropped IOL.

Amar Agarwal, MS, FRCS, FRCOphth is the Chairman and Managing Director of Dr. Agarwal's Group of Eye Hospitals and Eye Research Centre in India, which includes 97 hospitals worldwide; past President of the International Society of Refractive Surgery; and Secretary General of the Indian Intraocular Implant & Refractive Society.

Dr. Agarwal is the pioneer of phakonit, which is phacoemulsification with needle incision technology. This technique became popularly known as *bimanual phaco, microincision cataract surgery*, or *microphaco*. Dr. Agarwal was the first to remove cataracts through a 0.7-mm tip with the microphakonit technique. He also discovered no anesthesia cataract surgery and FAVIT (fallen vitreous), a new technique to remove dropped nuclei. Using an aquarium fish pump to increase the fluid into the eye in bimanual phaco and coaxial phaco has helped prevent surge. This formed the basis of various techniques of forced infusion for small-incision cataract surgery. Dr. Agarwal also discovered a new refractive error called *aberropia*. He was the first to perform a combined surgery of microphakonit (700-µm cataract surgery) with a 25-gauge vitrectomy in the same patient, thus creating the smallest incisions possible for cataract and vitrectomy. He was the first surgeon to implant a new mirror telescopic intraocular lens (IOL) for patients suffering from age-related macular degeneration. He was the first in the world to implant a glued IOL, in which a posterior chamber IOL is fixed in an eye without capsules using fibrin glue. He modified the Malyugin ring (MicroSurgical Technology) for small-pupil cataract surgery into the Agarwal modification of the Malyugin ring for miotic pupil cataract surgeries with posterior capsular defects.

Dr. Agarwal pioneered the technique of IOL scaffold, in which a 3-piece IOL is injected into an eye between the iris and the nucleus to prevent the nucleus from falling in posterior chamber ruptures. He combined glued IOL and IOL scaffold in cases of posterior chamber rupture where there is no iris or capsular support and termed the technique *glued IOL scaffold*. Pre-Descemet's endothelial keratoplasty was also pioneered by Dr. Agarwal. In this procedure, the pre-Descemet's layer and Descemet's membrane with endothelium are transplanted en bloc in patients with a diseased endothelium.

The first contact lens–assisted collagen cross-linking procedure, a new technique for cross-linking thin corneas, was performed in Dr. Agarwal's Eye Hospital, as were the first anterior segment transplantation in a 4-month-old patient with anterior staphyloma and the first glued endocapsular ring in cases of subluxated cataracts. Endoilluminator-assisted Descemet's membrane endothelial keratoplasty is also performed in Dr. Agarwal's Eye Hospital.

Dr. Agarwal has designed a new instrument for complicated cases called the *trocar anterior chamber maintainer*, which helps provide infusion through the anterior chamber and works like a trocar cannula. He has also started a new technique of iris suturing called *single-pass four-throw pupilloplasty*. This is used for closed-angle glaucoma, silicone oil-induced closed-angle glaucoma, and mydriatic cases. He has performed for the first time pinhole pupilloplasty to treat patients with astigmatism of up to 20 diopters.

Dr. Agarwal has performed more than 150 live surgeries at various conferences. His videos have won awards at the film festivals of the American Society of Cataract and Refractive Surgery, American Academy of Ophthalmology, and European Society of Cataract & Refractive Surgeons. He has written more than 75 books, which have been published in various languages, including English, Spanish, and Polish. He trains doctors from all over the world in his center on phaco, glued IOL, LASIK, and retinal surgeries.

The website of Dr. Agarwal's Eye Hospitals is www.dragarwal.com

Priya Narang, MS is Director of the Narang Eye Care & Laser Centre. In 1998, she earned her master of surgery in ophthalmology from B.J. Medical College in India.

Dr. Narang is a pioneer of the no-assistant technique for glued IOL. Her technique was published in the *Journal of Cataract & Refractive Surgery* in 2013 and was among the most-read top-5 articles for 2 quarters. She is also a pioneer of the widely accepted single-pass four-throw pupilloplasty technique that has various applications in the field of ophthalmology.

Dr. Narang has contributed many chapters and is an editor to various books published by top international publishers, including her latest book, *Optimizing Suboptimal Outcomes Following Cataract Surgery*. She is a reviewer to peer-reviewed journals, such as the *Indian Journal of Ophthalmology*. In 2016, she served as a consultant for the *Focal Point Module* at the American Academy of Ophthalmology. Her video blog on *Ocular Surgery News* features complex and challenging cataract cases.

In 2013, her paper "Glue-Assisted Intrascleral Fixation of Posterior Chamber Intraocular Lens" won the *Indian Journal of Ophthalmology*'s gold award for best paper. That same year, the Intraocular Implant & Refractive Society in India awarded her a gold medal for her contributions to the field of ophthalmology. For the past 3 years, her videos have been chosen for the Global Video Contest by the American Academy of Ophthalmology.

She is an internationally renowned speaker who regularly presents at the American Society of Cataract and Refractive Surgery, American Academy of Ophthalmology, World Ophthalmology Congress, and All India Ophthalmological Society.

Contributing Authors

Ashar Agarwal, MS, FRCS (Chapters 5 and 12)
Dr. Agarwal's Group of Eye Hospitals and Eye Research Centre
Chennai, India

Athiya Agarwal, MD, DO (Chapter 16)
Dr. Agarwal's Group of Eye Hospitals and Eye Research Centre
Chennai, India

Masayuki Akimoto, MD, PhD (Chapter 10 Case Presentation 2)
Osaka Red Cross Hospital
Osaka, Japan

Brandon D. Ayres, MD (Chapters 4 and 14)
Co-Director
Cornea Fellowship
Cornea Service
Wills Eye Hospital
Philadelphia, Pennsylvania

Sonal S. Chaugule, MS (Chapter 16)
Department of Ophthalmic Plastic Surgery, Orbit and Ocular Oncology
PBMA's H. V. Desai Eye Hospital
Pune, India

Robert J. Cionni, MD (Chapter 3 Case Presentation)
Director
Moran Eye Center
Department of Ophthalmology
University of Utah
The Eye Institute of Utah
Salt Lake City, Utah

Alan S. Crandall, MD (Chapter 2)
Moran Eye Center
University of Utah
Salt Lake City, Utah

Paul T. Finger, MD (Chapter 16)
Clinical Professor of Ophthalmology
Director
New York Eye Cancer Center
New York, New York

Sadeer B. Hannush, MD (Chapter 5 Case Presentation 2)
Attending Surgeon
Cornea Service
Wills Eye Hospital
Professor of Ophthalmology
Sidney Kimmel Medical College
Thomas Jefferson University
Medical Director
Lions Eye Bank of Delaware Valley
Philadelphia, Pennsylvania

Richard S. Hoffman, MD (Chapter 6)
Clinical Associate Professor of Ophthalmology
Casey Eye Institute
Oregon Health and Science University
Portland, Oregon

Santosh G. Honavar, MD, FACS, FRCOphth (Chapter 16)
Director
Ophthalmic Plastic Surgery and Ocular Oncology
Centre for Sight
Hyderabad, India

Dhivya Ashok Kumar, MD, FRCS, FICO, FAICO (Chapters 1 and 16)
Dr. Agarwal's Group of Eye Hospitals and Eye Research Centre
Chennai, India

Ravi Kumar K V, PGDO, FCO (LVPEI), FICO (SWISS) (Chapter 6 Case Presentation 2)
Former Chief Medical Officer
Rotary Eye Hospital
Vuyyuru, India

Mami Kusaka, MD (Chapter 10 Case Presentation 2)
Department of Ophthalmology and Visual Sciences
Graduate School of Medicine
Kyoto University
Kyoto, Japan

Yuri McKee, MD (Chapter 3)
East Valley Ophthalmology
Mesa, Arizona

Kevin M. Miller, MD (Chapter 9)
Kolokotrones Chair in Ophthalmology
Chief
Cataract and Refractive Surgery Division
Director
Anterior Segment Diagnostic Laboratory
David Geffen School of Medicine
University of California, Los Angeles
Stein Eye Institute
Los Angeles, California

Vladimir Pfeifer, MD, FEBOS-CR (Chapter 9 Case Presentation 3)
Chief
Cornea and Refractive Surgery Service
Head
Ljubljana Eye Bank
University Eye Hospital
Director
Eye Surgery Center
Ljubljana, Slovenia

Steven G. Safran, MD (Chapter 2 Case Presentation)
Capital Health System
Pennington, New Jersey
Penn Medicine Princeton Medical Center
Princeton, New Jersey
New Jersey Surgery Center
Mercerville, New Jersey

Michael E. Snyder, MD (Chapter 9 Case Presentation 2)
Clinical Governance Board Member
Chair
Clinical Research Steering Committee
Cincinnati Eye Institute
Professor of Ophthalmology
University of Cincinnati
Cincinnati, Ohio

William B. Trattler, MD (Foreword)
President
Center for Excellence in Eye Care
Volunteer Faculty
Florida International University College of Medicine
Miami, Florida

Claudio Trindade, MD, PhD (Chapter 15)
Board of Directors
Cançado-Trindade Eye Institute
Belo Horizonte, Brazil

David T. Truong, MD (Chapter 9)
Eye Associates of New Mexico
Albuquerque, New Mexico

Shin Yamane, MD, PhD (Chapter 8 Case Presentation 2)
Yamane Eye Clinic
Hiroshima, Japan

Preface

This book goes beyond basic teachings, presenting surgical knowledge that can help enhance surgical potential and avoid therapeutic missteps. Principles of surgical management of iris anomalies and defects are presented with the intention to help polish the arsenal of discreet medical and surgical facts.

The book is divided into 3 parts: Section I discusses the basics of various iris repair techniques; Section II features special topics that set a framework for managing iris repair; and Section III addresses the extended implications of iris repair. Each of the 16 chapters is abundantly referenced, presents evidence-based cases, and has video content. The case presentation in each chapter allows the reader to think further about the implications of surgical procedure and treatment.

The editors of this book have made extensive effort to ensure that the information is accurate and is useful to surgeons.

Ashvin Agarwal, MBBS, MS
Amar Agarwal, MS, FRCS, FRCOphth
Priya Narang, MS

Foreword

Mastering Iris Repair—the title describes exactly what readers can expect to achieve after reading the chapters and learning from the outstanding videos organized by 3 pioneers of this field. Surgical repair of the iris presents significant challenges to even experienced anterior segment surgeons. The editors, Ashvin Agarwal, MBBS, MS; Amar Agarwal, MS, FRCS, FRCOphth; and Priya Narang, MS, along with the contributing authors, have developed a curriculum of book chapters and videos that will enable surgeons to manage the iris with new insights and understanding. This is a must-read book for surgeons who want to excel in the area of iris repair.

The editors are gifted surgeons and educators. Dr. Narang and Dr. Amar Agarwal, in particular, have developed innovations that have profoundly impacted iris repair. They developed the single-pass four-throw pupilloplasty technique, which significantly simplifies surgical repair of the iris. Dr. Amar Agarwal also developed the pinhole pupilloplasty technique, which dramatically improves vision in patients with vision loss related to the cornea.

Beyond this book, the editors have helped me learn a variety of surgical skills that allow me to provide better care for my patients. Their vast experience in iris repair has been generously shared in many lectures that have taught surgeons the pearls and pitfalls of surgical repair of the iris.

The editors have invited world experts to contribute to the chapters and videos. These contributing authors make this an impressive book for young surgeons who want to learn more about surgical repair of the iris as well as experienced ophthalmic surgeons who would like to refine their skills to optimize surgery for their patients.

In summary, I would like to congratulate the editors for their hard work developing this extremely valuable book on iris repair. As ophthalmic surgeons, we will learn the variety of surgical techniques and tips to provide advanced surgical treatments for patients who require surgery on the iris.

William B. Trattler, MD

SECTION I

IRIS REPAIR TECHNIQUES

1

Introduction, Indications, and Salient Points of Iris Tissue and Repair

Dhivya Ashok Kumar, MD, FRCS, FICO, FAICO and Amar Agarwal, MS, FRCS, FRCOphth

Keywords

cerclage, iris repair, McCannel, pupilloplasty, Siepser technique, single-pass four-throw pupilloplasty, uvea

The pigmented iris tissue imparts the unique color to human eyes and is a part of the uvea, which is a highly vascular structure. The iris is a thin, soft structure that forms the entrance pathway, or pupil, through which light enters the eye. The iris tissue along with the lens acts as a vital diaphragm between the anterior and the posterior segments of the eye. The iris tissue can be injured in blunt or penetrating trauma causing subsequent iris defects. Congenital iris defects like coloboma or aniridia have also been reported. Being part of uveal tissue, it is antigenic and can also induce inflammation as it harbors pigment cells. Iris reconstruction and repair has been performed for various clinical conditions.[1-16] Iris reconstruction may fall broadly into 4 categories: optical (to improve quality of vision), functional (to improve visual acuity), structural (to reattach iris in its anatomical position), and cosmetic (to maintain pupil contour, iris color, and configuration). In this chapter, we will be highlighting the basics of applied anatomy, history, common repair principles, and key points of iris repair.

Anatomy of the Iris

The iris is the anteriormost part of the uvea that forms a thin circular diaphragm dividing the eye into anterior and posterior chambers. Its diameter is around 12 mm, while its thickness varies.[1] It is thinnest at its root, where it is attached to the anterior surface of the ciliary body, and

Agarwal A, Agarwal A, eds. *Mastering Iris Repair: A Video Textbook of Iris Repair and Pupilloplasty Techniques* (pp 3-12).

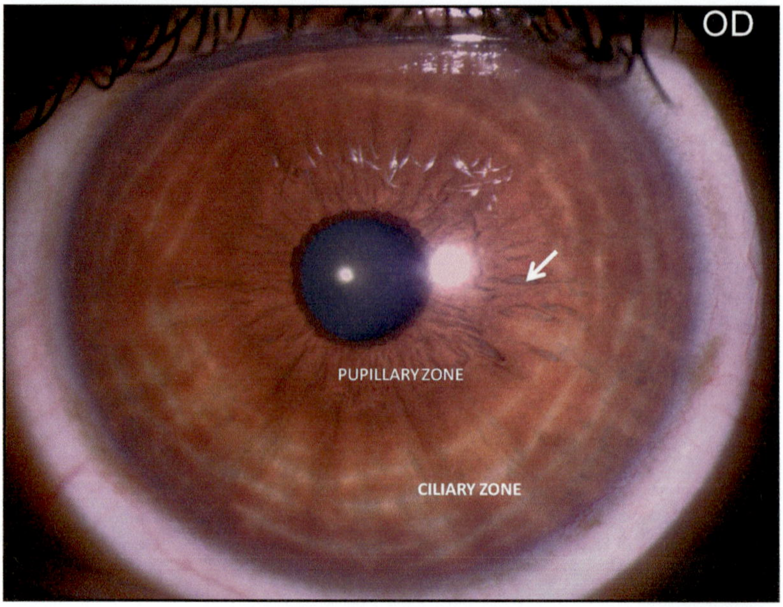

Figure 1-1. Clinical image showing the normal architecture of iris (arrow indicates crypts).

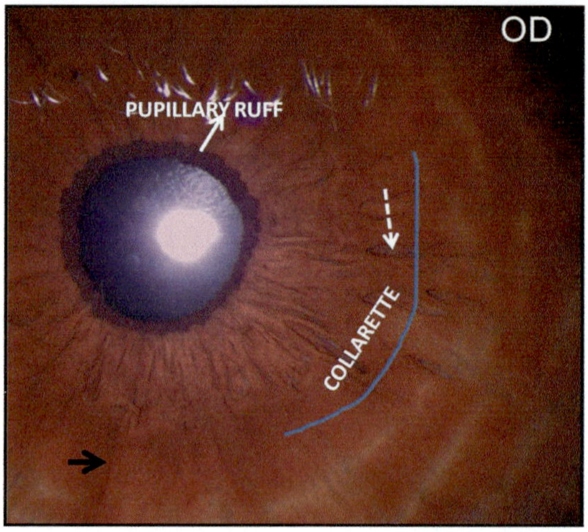

Figure 1-2. High magnification image of iris showing collarette (blue line), furrows (black arrow), Fuch's crypts (white dotted arrow), and pupillary frill or ruff (white arrow).

thickest at about 2 mm from the pupillary margin, where it is called the *collarette* (Figure 1-1).[1] The collarette divides the anterior surface of the iris into 2 zones—the ciliary zone and pupillary zone. The ciliary zone has a velvety surface with characteristic radial streaks, crypts, and contraction furrows (Figure 1-2). The radial streaks are trabeculae, or bands of connective tissue, formed by radiating blood vessels from the major arterial circle. A few oval-shaped depressions, called Fuch's crypts, are more pronounced near the collarette. They are enclosed by the bands of radial streaks. Contraction furrows are concentric lines around the collarette that are more visible when the pupil dilates. The pupillary zone is relatively smooth and flat except at the pupillary border where the iris posterior pigmented epithelium extends slightly anteriorly to form the pupillary frill. The posterior surface of the iris is dark with multiple radial contraction folds and circular furrows.

Histology of the Iris

The iris consists of an anterior limiting layer, stromal layer, anterior epithelial layer, and posterior pigmented epithelial layer. The anterior limiting layer is a thin, condensed part of anterior stroma. It is absent in areas with crypts. The stromal layer forms the bulk of the iris tissue. It is a highly vascularized layer that consists of collagen fibers, fibroblasts, melanocytes, nerve fibers, and pupillary muscles in a mucopolysaccharide matrix. The radial vessels branching from the major arterial circle form an incomplete minor arterial circle of iris at the collarette. The iris vessels are lined by non-fenestrated endothelium and are devoid of internal elastic lamina. The anterior epithelial layer lies underneath the stroma. It has relatively fewer melanin granules. It is the anterior continuation of the outer pigmented layer of ciliary epithelium. The posterior epithelial layer consists of cuboidal cells that are packed with melanin granules and are, hence, heavily pigmented. This layer is a continuation of the inner nonpigmented layer of ciliary epithelium.

Pupil Anatomy

The pupil is a circular aperture in the iris that limits the amount of light reaching the retina. It is situated slightly nasally. The margins of the pupil have a pigment frill called the *pupillary ruff* (see Figure 1-2) formed by a slight anterior extension of the posterior pigmented layer. Two intrinsic pupillary muscles, present in the iris stromal layer, control the size of the pupil according to the intensity of the incident light. One is the circumferential sphincter pupillae muscle supplied by the parasympathetic nervous system. It is present in the pupillary zone of the iris forming a circular band of about 1 mm in size. It constricts the pupil. Another is the radial dilator pupillae muscle supplied by the sympathetic system. It is situated in the ciliary zone of the iris. It dilates the pupil. The normal pupillary diameter varies from 2 to 4 mm in bright light and 4 to 8 mm in dim light.[1] In most individuals, pupils are generally equal in size. However, in 25% of normal subjects, the pupils differ slightly in size.[1] The size and shape of the pupil can be altered due to congenital, neurological, pharmacological, traumatic, and surgical causes.

Iris and Pupillary Abnormalities

Iris sphincter tears causing traumatic mydriasis and iridodialysis causing a distorted pupil are common following contusive trauma to the eye. Penetrating trauma to the eye can also cause damage to the iris. A damaged or irreversibly dilated pupil can result in bothersome glare and photophobia limiting the visual functions of the eye. A pupil with abnormal shape or size is also cosmetically unappealing. Hence, a procedure that reconstructs the iris and pupil to near normal shape, size, and position is of substantial benefit. Iridoplasty is the surgical method of reconstructing the injured or defective iris. Pupilloplasty is a surgical procedure designed to reconstruct a pupil that has an altered configuration due to an irreversible cause. The procedure has been popular for many decades.

Indications for Iris Repair

The indications for iris reconstruction and pupilloplasty include the following:

- Congenital iris defects like coloboma of the iris (Figure 1-3), aniridia (Figure 1-4), and polycoria
- Traumatic mydriasis (Figure 1-5)
- Neurogenic mydriasis
- Traumatic iris defects and iridodialysis (Figure 1-6)
- Iatrogenic iris injuries due to surgical trauma
- Urrets-Zavalia syndrome
- Pinhole pupil optics
- Iridoplasty for angle-closure glaucoma (ACG)
- To reconstruct the iris before endothelial keratoplasty

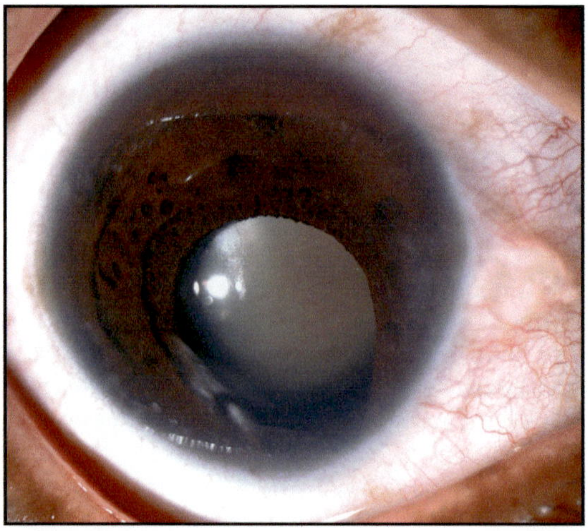

Figure 1-3. Clinical image showing the inferior iris coloboma with cataract.

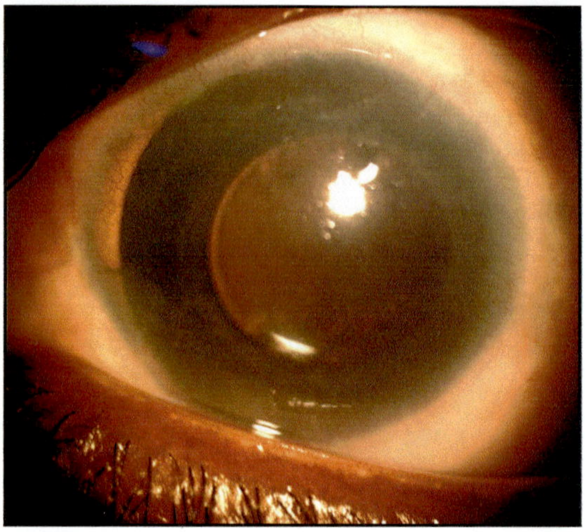

Figure 1-4. Congenital aniridia with aniridia intraocular lens (IOL) in situ.

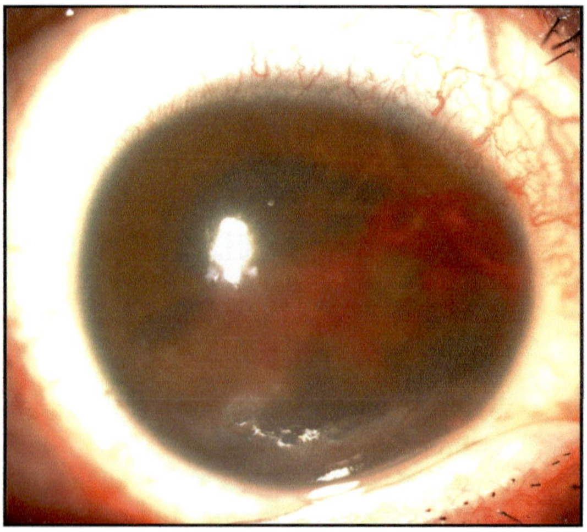

Figure 1-5. Traumatic mydriasis following blunt ocular trauma.

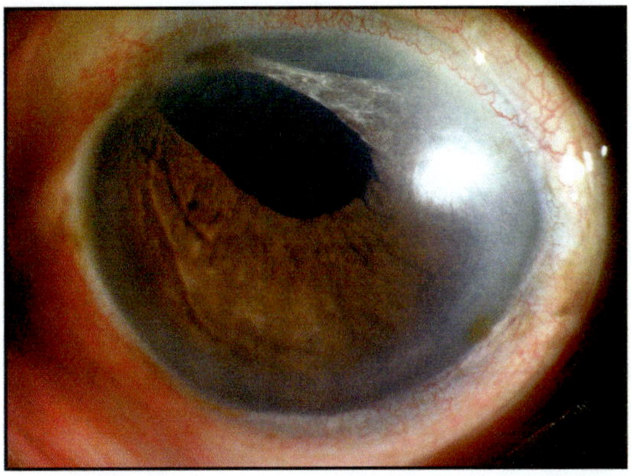

Figure 1-6. Post-traumatic iridodialysis in a pseudophakic eye.

History and Techniques

McCannel was the first to introduce the concept of using a monofilament suture within a contained anterior chamber to correct iridodialysis.[3] In 1976, McCannel originally used a curved needle for his iris suture technique for iris reconstruction. Later modifications and innovations led to the development of the 17-mm straight McCannel needle with 10-0 polypropylene sutures.[4] However, in the McCannel suture technique, the iris leaflets, along with the suture, need to be brought out of the limbal stab incision to tie the knot. Though the technique proved promising for peripheral iris defects and iridodialysis clefts, a larger defect or a more central involvement demanded more intraoperative manipulation and iris traction.

The single suture loop pupilloplasty, explained by Behndig,[5] involved 3 corneal stab incisions and the use of a slightly bent PC-7 needle (Alcon) with 10-0 polypropylene suture that, he believed, was easy to maneuver inside the closed anterior chamber. However, the procedure involves passage of the needle through multiple contiguous points on the iris, near the pupillary border, to form a continuous row of sutures in between the 3 stab incisions. The 2 suture ends are retrieved through the first stab incision and tied and the knot is internalized into the anterior chamber. Ogawa[6] described a conceptually similar technique, called *iris cerclage*, in the same year for postoperative atonic pupil. Nevertheless, both procedures involved meticulous and technically challenging manipulations within the anterior chamber. Thus, the chances of intraoperative complications increased with all these procedures.

The Siepser sliding knot technique and its modifications proved invaluable in reducing the chances of intraoperative complications.[7,8] The technique involves 2 limbal stab incisions. A long needle with 9-0 or 10-0 polypropylene suture is advanced through 1 stab incision, passed through the proximal and distal iris leaflets and then retrieved out with the help of a cannula inserted through another stab incision. A microhook is used to retrieve a loop of the distal part of the suture through the first stab incision. Two throws are made by passing the trailing end of the suture down through the loop. The suture ends are gently pulled so that the suture knot slips inside, drawing the iris leaflets together. The distal suture loop is again retrieved through the stab incision. Siepser sliding knot involves passing the trailing end of suture twice from below upward through the second loop. Osher et al[8] suggested passing the trailing end once through the loop from below upwards, directing it under the trailing strand and then pulling the suture ends to slide the locking knot. A conceptually and technically simplified procedure called single-pass four-throw pupilloplasty (SFT), that ensures the formation of a non-loosening knot with minimal manipulation of the iris tissue was introduced by Narang and Agarwal.[9] This technique is a variation of the modified Siepser slip-knot technique. It involves retrieving a loop of suture from the distal end, in a similar fashion, as is done in the modified Siepser slip-knot technique. One can also make the pupil into a pinhole with this method so that astigmatism problems are solved (Videos 1-1 and 1-2). Instead of passing the proximal suture-end twice through the loop, this technique involves 4 throws through the loop (Figure 1-7). The helical knot is then made to slip into the anterior chamber. The procedure can be repeated on other areas of the iris to fashion a round, smaller sized pupil.

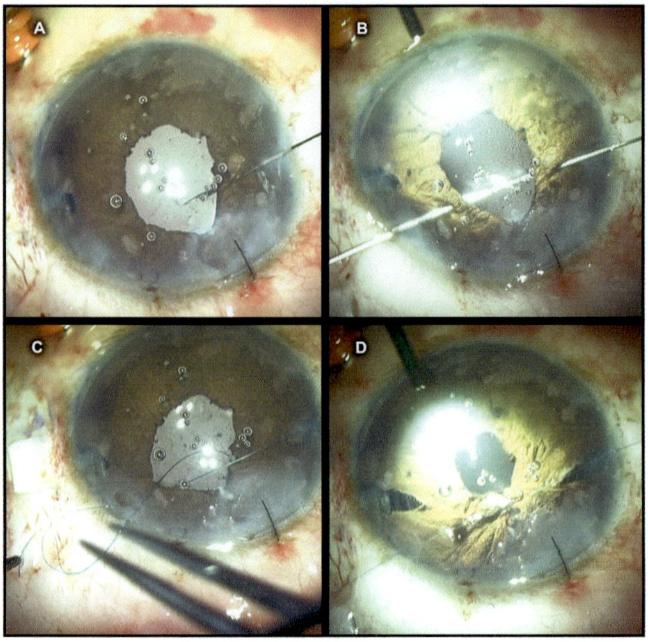

Figure 1-7. SFT. (A) Side port made and 10-0 Prolene (Ethicon) suture inserted into the iris leaflet on one end. (B) Suture needle passed through the other side of the iris. (C) Suture loop formed, pulled out, and 4 throws passed through it. (D) Knot tightened and slid into the anterior chamber followed by incision of the suture ends.

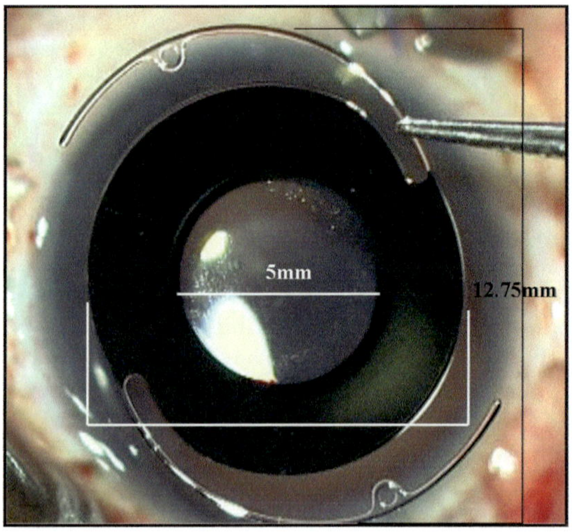

Figure 1-8. Glued iris prosthesis implant for total aniridia with absent capsules.

In cases with extensive tissue loss, it may not be possible to reconfigure the whole iris. In such situations, an iris prosthetic implant may be used. Iris color and configuration can be decided according to the needs of the patient. In eyes with small defects of the iris with intact capsule, a segmental iris prosthesis can be used. In eyes with a total iris defect, an aniridia implant is preferred (Figure 1-8). In eyes with aniridia with loss of capsules, a glued iris prosthesis can be used.[10]

Salient Points in Iris Tissue Repair

- The basic principle in iris tissue repair is to reconstruct the anatomical position and retain the contour and configuration for a positive functional and cosmetic outcome.
- Preoperative workup can include clinical photography, anterior segment optical coherence tomography (AS-OCT; Figure 1-9), and microscopy (contraindicated in traumatic cases).
- The key step in iris defect repair is to appose the flaps of iris without excess crowding or tissue loss.

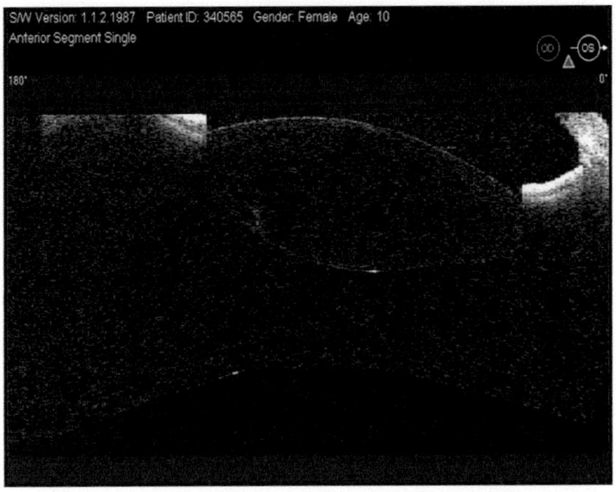

Figure 1-9. AS-OCT showing partial aniridia with cataractous lens.

- The vital step in any pupilloplasty procedure is to tie a locking knot that prevents slippage of the sutures and keeps the iris leaflets apposed.
- The technicality in creating the locking knot is what determines the intricacy of the procedure.
- The objective in iris repair involving the pupil is to form a round and central pupil. Large pupils will lead to abnormal glare and visual dysphotopsia while small pupils will restrict visual acuity by diffraction; therefore, aiming for optimum pupil size is critical. While centering the pupil position intraoperatively, it is important to look at the position of the corneal vertex, or Purkinje image, to center the papillary axis.
- The objective in iris dialysis repair is to reattach the iris root in the specific region.
- It is vital to keep the anterior chamber formed intraoperatively throughout the procedure of iris repair by using a viscoelastic device.
- An anterior chamber maintainer can be used to maintain chamber stability. An air pump–assisted anterior chamber maintainer can help in tamponade of inadvertent intraoperative hyphema.[11]
- Nonabsorbable suture material, either 9-0 or 10-0 polypropylene, is preferred for iris suturing.
- Minimizing tissue handling and manipulation can help prevent excessive pigment release and thereby reduce postoperative inflammation.
- Releasing the intraocular adhesions of the iris is crucial before initiating iris repair.
- Iris prolapse for long duration has to be abscised to prevent transfer of microbial agents and subsequent infection.

Advantages of Iris Repair

Iris defect repair can help reduce photophobia and glare by decreasing the pupillary size. The procedure also decreases intraocular pressure in patients with appositional angle closure as in cases of primary ACG, chronic ACG, plateau iris syndrome, failed laser peripheral iridotomies, and Urrets-Zavalia syndrome (Figure 1-10).[12] There are other reported indications of SFT. In endothelial keratoplasty, performing a pupilloplasty helps to compartmentalize the eye into anterior and posterior chambers, thus maintaining adequate air pressure in the anterior chamber to enable attachment of the graft.[13] The pupilloplasty procedure is also useful in preventing optic capture and tilting of IOLs in case of glued intrascleral fixation of the IOL.[14] Narrowing the pupil to the size of a pinhole is considered a pinhole pupilloplasty. The pinhole effect blocks distorted and unfocused light rays and focuses the rays through the central aperture. This reduces aberrations of the optical system and enhances visual acuity (see Video 1-2). A recent study has shown pinhole optics by pupilloplasty procedure improving visual outcomes in patients with corneal astigmatism.[15]

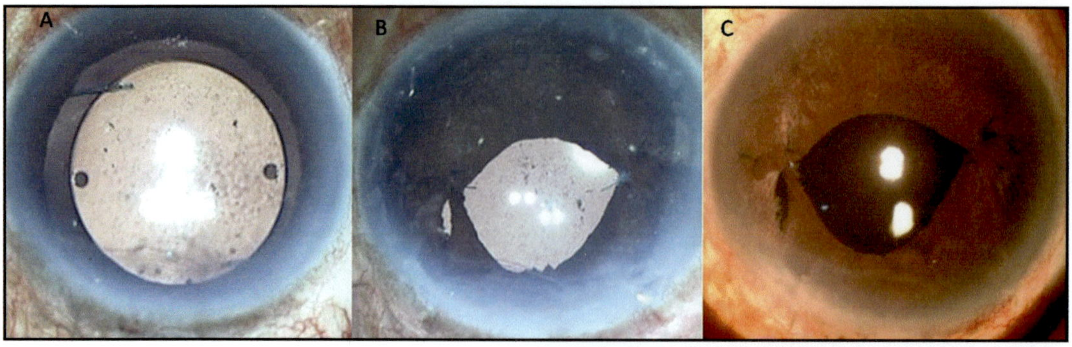

Figure 1-10. (A) Urrets-Zavalia syndrome. (B) Postoperative day 1. (C) One month following SFT.

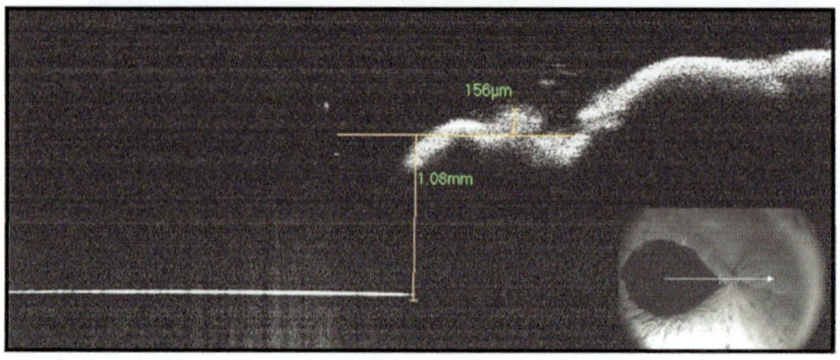

Figure 1-11. Spectral domain optical coherence tomography analysis of iris showing the elevated knot complex above the iris plane.

Imaging of Iris Knot

AS-OCT can be used for direct visualization of suture knots after pupilloplasty (Figure 1-11). In a recent study on pupilloplasty knot evaluation, we measured the length and position of knots using spectral domain optical coherence tomography.[16] The following can be measured: length of suture cut ends, position from the corneal endothelium, iris configuration, tethering, and pupil size.

Discussion

Iris repair has been popular for more than 3 decades; however, because of the unique structural and functional features of the iris, not many surgeons develop the delicate surgical skills necessary to manage its complications. Nevertheless, in the last 2 decades there have been many improvements in techniques resulting in improved anatomical, functional, and cosmetic outcomes in iris reconstruction. Identifying the exact etiology and addressing the needs of individual patients is of the utmost importance in the selection of iris repair procedure.

Case Presentation

Cigarette Lighter Injury

Dhivya Ashok Kumar, MD, FRCS, FICO, FAICO and
Amar Agarwal, MS, FRCS, FRCOphth

A young male presented with a history of a cigarette lighter bursting in his face. The lens, cornea, and iris were damaged. The corneal tear repair was done elsewhere. We performed a lensectomy with a glued IOL. The iridodialysis was repaired using the hang-back technique. The pupil was decentered so we used the vitrectomy probe to create a pupil in the area where the corneal scar was not present. The patient's vision improved to 6/9 (Figure 1-12 and Video 1-3).

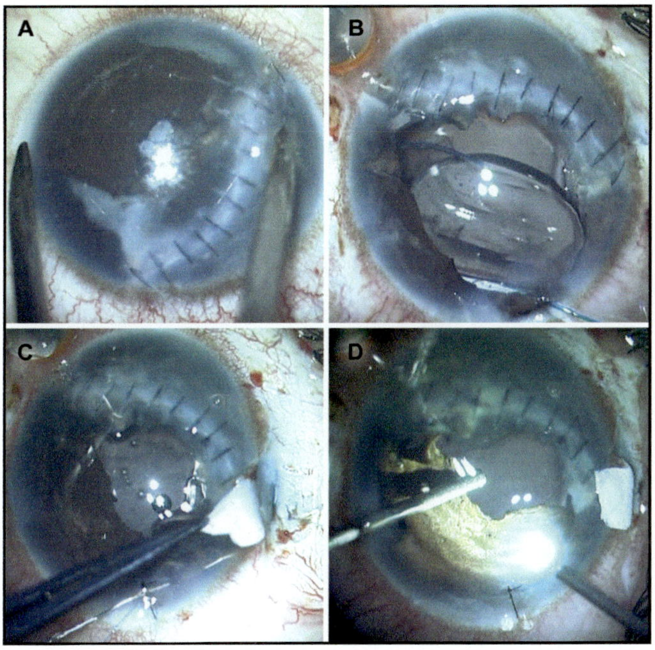

Figure 1-12. SFT surgical technique. (A) Cigarette lighter injury in a young male. Note the corneal tear repair done elsewhere. The lens and iris are damaged. (B) Lensectomy is performed followed by a glued IOL surgery. (C) Double-armed Prolene suture is used to perform the hang-back technique to fix the iridodialysis. (D) The vitrectomy probe helps create a pupil away from the corneal scar. The patient had 6/9 vision postoperatively.

References

1. Snell RS, Lemp MA. *Clinical Anatomy of the Eye*. Hoboken, NJ: Blackwell Science; 1998:165-166.
2. Remington LA. *Clinical Anatomy of the Visual System*. Maryland Heights, MO: Elsevier; 2005:41.
3. McCannel MA. A retrievable suture idea for anterior uveal problems. *Ophthalmic Surg Lasers Imaging Retina*. 1976;7(2):98-99.
4. Nunziata BR. Repair of iridodialysis using a 17-millimeter straight needle. *Ophthalmic Surg*. 1993;24:627-629.
5. Behndig A. Small incision single-suture-loop pupilloplasty for postoperative atonic pupil. *J Cataract Refract Surg*. 1998;24:1429-1431.
6. Ogawa GS. The iris cerclage suture for permanent mydriasis: a running suture technique. *Ophthalmic Surg Lasers Imaging Retina*. 1998;29(12):1001-1009.
7. Siepser SB. The closed chamber slipping suture technique for iris repair. *Ann Ophthalmol*. 1994;26:71-72.
8. Osher RH, Snyder ME, Cionni RJ. Modification of the Siepser slip-knot technique. *J Cataract Refract Surg*. 2005;31(6):1098-1100.
9. Narang P, Agarwal A. Single-pass four-throw technique for pupilloplasty. *Eur J Ophthalmol*. 2017;27(4):506-508.
10. Kumar DA, Agarwal A, Prakash G, Jacob S. Managing total aniridia with aphakia using a glued iris prosthesis. *J Cataract Refract Surg*. 2010;36(5):864-865.
11. Agarwal A, Narang P, Kumar DA, Agarwal A. Trocar anterior chamber maintainer: improvised infusion technique. *J Cataract Refract Surg*. 2016;42(2):185-189.
12. Narang P, Agarwal A, Kumar DA. Single-pass four-throw pupilloplasty for angle-closure glaucoma. *Indian J Ophthalmol*. 2018;66(1):120.
13. Narang P, Agarwal A, Kumar DA. Single-pass 4-throw pupilloplasty for pre-Descemet endothelial keratoplasty. *Cornea*. 2017;36(12):1580-1583.
14. Narang P, Agarwal A. Glued intrascleral haptic fixation of an intraocular lens. *Indian J Ophthalmol*. 2017;65(12):1370.
15. Narang P, Agarwal A, Ashok Kumar D, Agarwal A. Pinhole pupilloplasty: small-aperture optics for higher-order corneal aberrations. *J Cataract Refract Surg*. 2019;45(5):539-543.
16. Kumar DA, Agarwal A, Chandrasekar R, Jaganathasamy N. Iris and knot configuration after single pass four throw (SFT) pupilloplasty as imaged by the spectral-domain optical coherence tomography. *Indian J Ophthalmol*. 2019;67(2):209-212.

Please visit www.routledge.com/9781630917265

to access additional material.

2

Mastering the McCannel Suture and Modified McCannel Suture Techniques

Alan S. Crandall, MD

Keywords

iris reconstruction, iris repair, McCannel, modified McCannel, Siepser sliding knot, single-pass four-throw pupilloplasty

Iris defects can be managed by various surgical interventions that may involve alterations to the cornea, including corneal tattooing. Additionally, it may also involve reconstruction or manipulation of the iris, or insertion of an opaque ring in the lenticular plane. The decision of which approach may be most beneficial depends on a variety of factors that include the area of iris defect present and positioning of iris defect–associated dysfunctional abnormalities, like iris chaffing or transillumination defects. Functional and structural abnormalities and variations, like presence of synechiae, which that can be either anterior or posterior, should also be considered.

Trauma, including surgical, can cause the following 5 types of iris defects:

1. Iris holes
2. Sphincter tears
3. Iridodialysis
4. Partial or total iris loss
5. Traumatic mydriasis

A congenital coloboma or peripheral iris defect can be repaired at the time of cataract extraction using the same surgical principals. For the iris repair, it is important to use a suture material that is not biodegradable. Both 9-0 and 10-0 polypropylene (Prolene, Ethicon) are available on a number of different needles. Understanding the properties of the needles and the configuration is necessary to perform the repair. When passing the needle, it is important to make sure that corneal

Agarwal A, Agarwal A, eds. *Mastering Iris Repair: A Video Textbook of Iris Repair and Pupilloplasty Techniques* (pp 13-19).

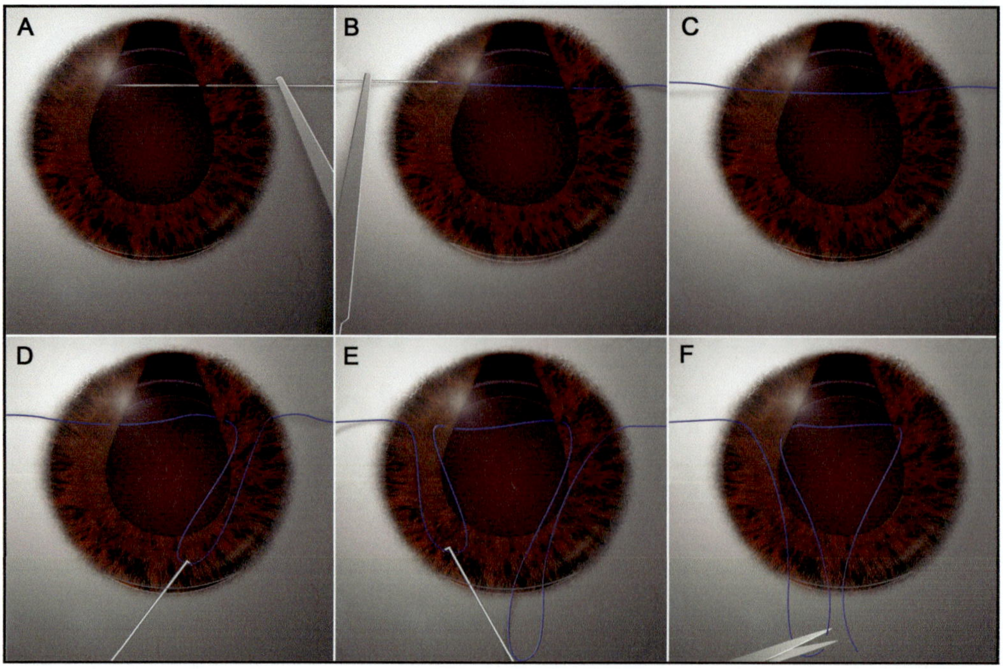

Figure 2-1. Part 1: Illustration depicting modified McCannel suturing. (A) 10-0 Prolene suture with straight needle passed through the cornea and iris. (B) Suture and needle passed through the other end of the iris and cornea. (C) Suture from one end of the iris to the other. (D) One end of the loop of suture brought out through the clear corneal incision. (E) The other loop is also brought out through the clear corneal incision. (F) Suture ends that are seen outside the clear corneal incision are cut. (Reprinted with permission from Dr. Agarwal's Eye Hospital and Eye Research Centre.)

tissue is not caught. Use a gentle back-and-forth movement of the needle as it is passed through the paracenteses to ensure no corneal stroma or Descemet's membrane is caught.

A McCannel suture[1] is most suitable to close an iris defect through a paracentesis if the defect is peripheral. McCannel[1] originally described the repair of iridodialysis with a 10-0 nylon suture on a curved needle. To close larger central defects, use either a Siepser sliding knot[2] or the newer technique of single-pass four-throw pupilloplasty developed by Narang and Agarwal.[3,4]

Surgical Technique

All iris repair procedures are performed under peribulbar anesthesia, and supplemental anesthesia is provided, as necessary, depending upon the surgical scenario.

McCannel Suture

The original McCannel technique involves creation of 2 paracentesis incisions at the limbus on the sides opposite to each other at either end of the iris defect. After inflating the anterior chamber with adequate viscoelastic, a long, thin needle with a 10-0 polypropylene suture is introduced through the paracentesis site. The needle is then passed through the proximal and distal edge of the iris defect. A corneal incision is created between the 2 paracentesis incisions, the iris tissue is pulled out, and the sutures tied. The iris tissue is then reposited inside the anterior chamber.

Modified McCannel Suture

The modified McCannel suture is a closed chamber approach[5] wherein the suture is withdrawn from the corneal incision and the knot is tied externally without pulling the iris tissue from the corneal incision (Figures 2-1 through 2-5 and Video 2-1). This knot is then slid inside the anterior chamber and end-opening forceps are introduced through the paracentesis incision, which help to

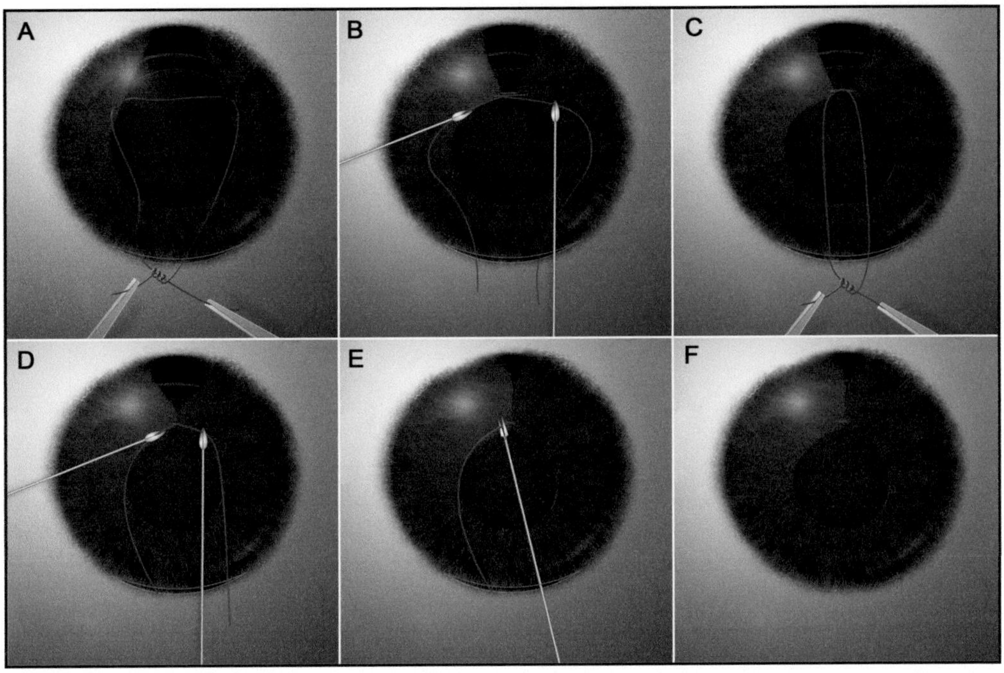

Figure 2-2. Part 2: Illustration depicting modified McCannel suturing. (A) Three throws placed between the sutures. (B) Throws passed into the anterior chamber. Two microforceps used to tie the knot. (C) Another throw put between the sutures creating the knot. (D) Two microforceps used to tie the knot. (E) Microscissors cut the suture ends. (F) Case completed. Iris coloboma sutured with the modified McCannel technique. (Reprinted with permission from Dr. Agarwal's Eye Hospital and Eye Research Centre.)

approximate the edges of the iris defect, to fix the suture knot. This maneuver is repeated as many times as needed for adequate closure of an iris defect.

Discussion

When approaching an eye with iris damage it is important to understand that there will likely be adhesions that must be freed in order to reconstruct a functional eye. Most adhesions to the lens (natural or pseudophakic) tend to be at the sphincter and can be released with blunt dissection with a cyclodialysis spatula or the cannula on the viscoelastic syringe. If the adhesions are extensive, then the use of intraocular scissors may be required. It is also important to know if peripheral anterior synechiae (PAS) are present and their location. Gonioscopy prior to surgery, or the use of an intraoperative gonioscopic lens, such as the direct or indirect Ahmed Gonio Lens (Ocular Instruments, Inc), is necessary to identify the extent of the PAS and to game plan. The PAS can usually be released using microforceps or gentle blunt dissection with the cyclodialysis spatula. Freeing PAS can lead to an easier repair by making the iris more mobile and more tissue available. Occasionally, after the iris repair, the pupil may be slightly decentered or too small, requiring iris sphincterotomies.

Large iris defects or total loss of the iris may require the use of an artificial iris device. Morcher makes devices with a variety of configurations that can help with light scattering, but they are black and, as a result, not cosmetically pleasing. Although not US Food and Drug Administration–approved, these devices can be obtained with a compassionate-use exemption. The only Food and Drug Administration–approved artificial iris is the CustomFlex Artificial Iris (HumanOptics).

To repair an iridodialysis, a double-armed mattress suture technique is used. I usually use straight needles and pass the needle 1.5 mm posterior to the scleral spur and rotate the knot into the sclera to prevent discomfort and late erosion. If the defect is large, use another mattress suture or the sewing machine technique.[6]

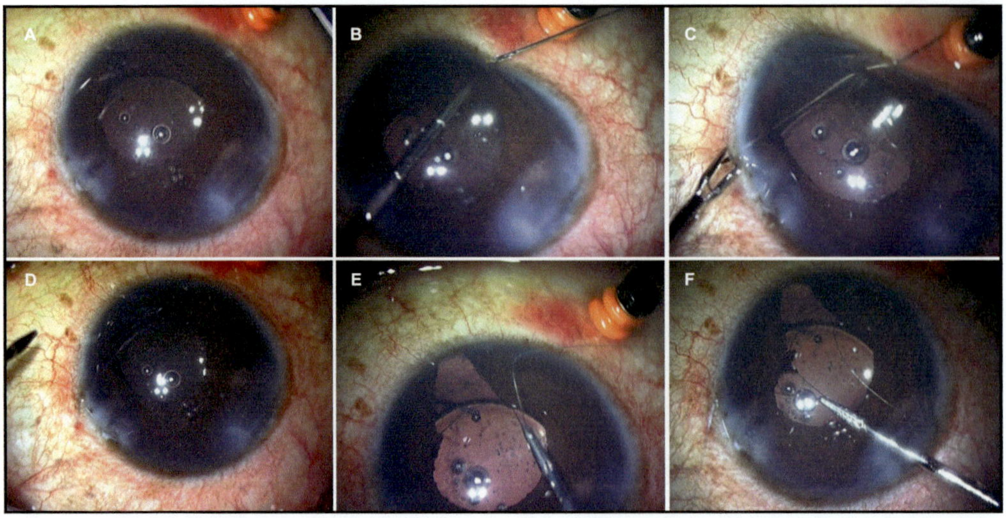

Figure 2-3. Part 1: Modified McCannel suturing. (A) Iris coloboma. (B) 10-0 Prolene suture with straight needle passed through the cornea and iris. (C) Suture and needle passed through the other end of the iris and cornea. (D) Suture brought out. (E) One end of the loop of suture brought out through the clear corneal incision. (F) Other loop is also brought out through the clear corneal incision. (Reprinted with permission from Dr. Agarwal's Eye Hospital and Eye Research Centre.)

Pupil Repair

Blunt injury can cause permanent sphincter damage that should be repaired at the time of cataract surgery, because the surgery will likely uncover light scattering or visual disturbances that may not have been noticed prior to surgery. The patient can also develop dysphotopsia from peripheral intraocular lens exposure. Following intraocular surgery, permanent sphincter damage can be caused by Urrets-Zavalia syndrome.[7] Two techniques can be used to repair this condition.

A pupillary cerclage (a 360-degree purse string) is an elegant technique. If performing a cerclage at the time of cataract surgery, 2 or 3 additional paracenteses will be required. If the repair is done following cataract/intraocular lens surgery, then 4 paracenteses will be needed. Use a 10-0 Prolene suture on a CTC-6L (Ethicon) or a PC-7 (Alcon) needle. You can start the cerclage through the main incision. The needle is passed in and out of the iris (mid-periphery rather than at the sphincter) usually 3 to 4 times and then docked into a cannula (I generally use the viscoelastic cannula) before it is removed. It is important to remember that because the needle is curved care must be used to avoid hitting the cornea or the lens. This process is repeated until the full 360 degrees of the iris is completed. The knot is then tied through the main incision after the pupil is constricted to 3.5 to 4 mm. The needle is passed through the iris mid-periphery versus the sphincter to avoid pulling the suture into the pupil when constricting the pupil and erosion over time.

Another option, that is just as functional, is to use multiple (3 or 4) interrupted sutures. The result is a square- or diamond-shaped pupil. This much simpler technique requires 3 or 4 paracenteses with Siepser or single-pass four-throw knots. Although the result is not as cosmetically pleasing, a few of the knots in the multiple interrupted sutures can be cut if, at some point, the patient needs a larger pupil. If this is attempted with the cerclage technique, the pupil may end up too large.

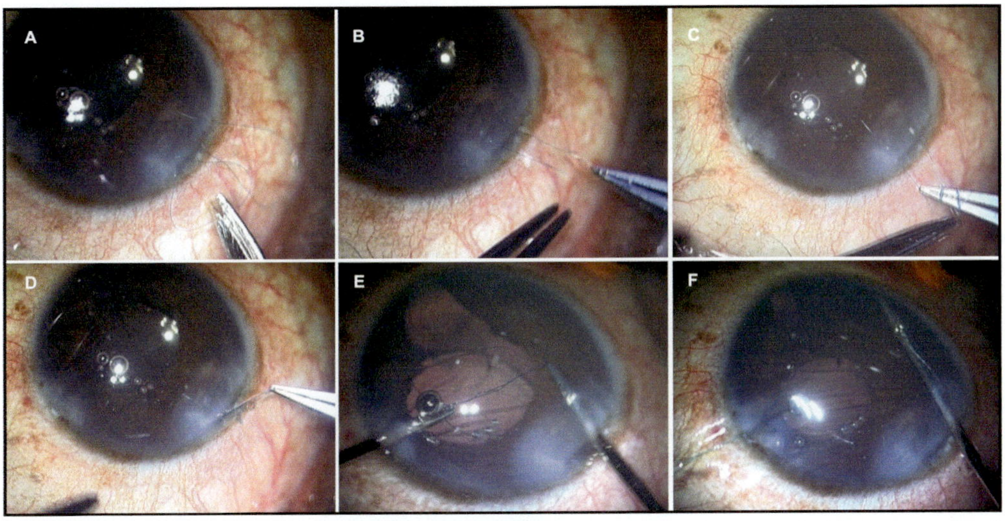

Figure 2-4. Part 2: Modified McCannel suturing. (A) Suture ends are cut. (B) Throws made. (C) Knot completed. One can make 3-2-1 throws. (D) Throws passed into the anterior chamber. (E) Two microforceps used to tie the knot. (F) Knot completed. (Reprinted with permission from Dr. Agarwal's Eye Hospital and Eye Research Centre.)

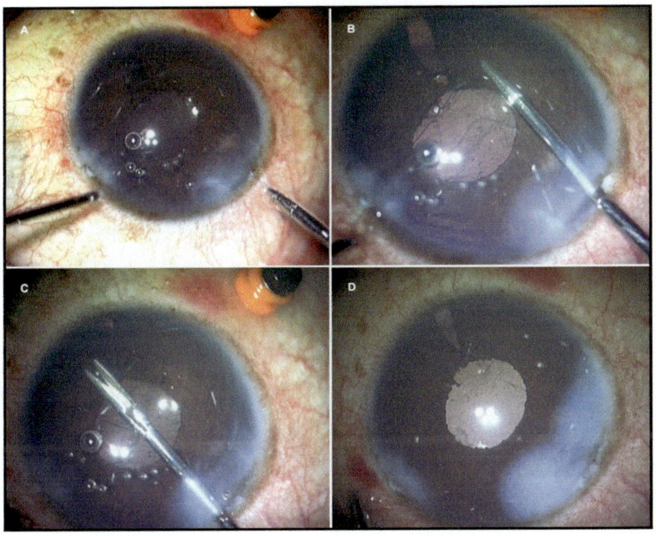

Figure 2-5. Part 3: Modified McCannel suturing. (A) Same process repeated. (B) Knot tied with the microforceps in a 3-2-1 fashion. (C) Microscissors cut the suture ends. (D) Case completed. Iris coloboma sutured with the modified McCannel technique. (Reprinted with permission from of Dr. Agarwal's Eye Hospital and Eye Research Centre.)

Case Presentation

Modified McAhmed Suture Technique

Steven G. Safran, MD

A patient who has an iris defect can be sutured using the McCannel technique. Another method is the modified McAhmed technique of iris suturing, called the McAhmed suture technique. In this method, a 10-0 Prolene suture is used. The entire suture is pulled out on one side and then brought into the anterior chamber and tied. This can be performed using microforceps (Figure 2-6 and Video 2-2).

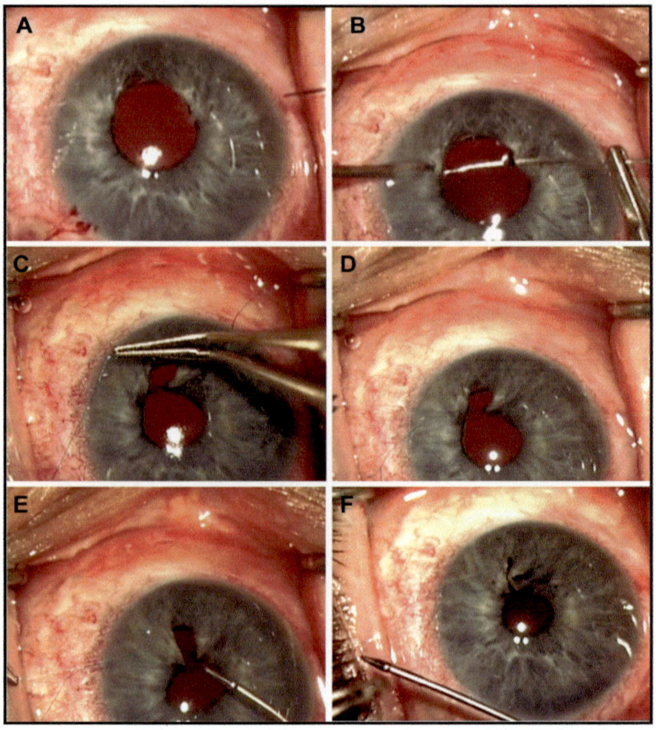

Figure 2-6. Modified McAhmed suture technique. (A) Iris defect. **(B)** 10-0 Prolene suture passed through the iris. (C) Suture brought out to one side. (D) Suture tied outside the eye. (E) Suture brought inside the anterior chamber. (F) Iris repair done.

References

1. McCannel MA. A retrieval suture idea for anterior uveal problems. *Ophthalmic Surg.* 1976;7(2):98-103
2. Siepser SB. The closed chamber slipping suture technique for iris repair. *Ann Ophthalmol.* 1994;26:71-72
3. Narang P, Agarwal A. Single-pass four-throw technique for pupilloplasty. *Eur J Ophthalmol.* 2017;27:506-508.
4. Narang P, Agarwal A, Agarwal A, Agarwal A. Twofold technique of non-appositional repair with single-pass four-throw pupilloplasty for iridodialysis. *J Cataract Refract Surg.* 2018;44:1413-1420.
5. Blackmon DM, Lambert SR. Congenital iris coloboma repair using a modified McCannel suture technique. *Am J Ophthalmol.* 2003;135(5):730-732.
6. Silva JL, Povoa J, Lobo C, Murta J. New technique for iridodialysis correction: single-knot sewing-machine suture. *J Cataract Refract Surg.* 2016;42:520-523.
7. Spierer O, Lazar M. Urrets-Zavalia syndrome (fixed and dilated pupil following penetrating keratoplasty for keratoconus) and its variants. *Surv Ophthalmol.* 2014;59(3):304-310.

Please visit www.routledge.com/9781630917265

to access additional material.

3

Mastering the Siepser Iris Suture Technique

Yuri McKee, MD and Ashvin Agarwal, MBBS, MS

Keywords

iris repair, modified Siepser, Siepser technique, single-pass four-throw pupilloplasty

The ability to pass a sliding knot into the eye via a small incision is a critical skill for ophthalmic surgeons. Iris repair, coloboma repair, iris cerclage, iridodialysis repair, intraocular lens (IOL) fixation, or fixation of intraocular hardware are all examples of surgical procedures where introducing a sliding knot through a small corneal incision can help maintain a closed anterior chamber thereby increasing surgical safety. The original description of the technique by Siepser,[1] and the subsequent modifications of the technique by Osher et al.,[2] primarily deal with repair of the iris (Videos 3-1 and 3-2).

Materials

For suture material that is to be passed through the iris, a 10-0 or 9-0 polypropylene material is preferred. For the Siepser technique, a long, curved needle (CIF-4, Ethicon) or long, straight needle (STC-6, Ethicon) is required. The suture should not be double-armed. Adequate suture length should be ensured to allow for tension-free maneuvers while repairing iris defects. Surgical instruments should include a 1-mm paracentesis blade, a 27-gauge cannula, a fine locking needle driver, a set of trying forceps, fine intraocular forceps, and intraocular scissors, and a small hook suitable for intraocular suture retrieval. The hook for suture removal can be a Kuglen hook, Sinskey hook, Shepard hook, a Condon snare, or any small hook that can easily fit through a paracentesis to retrieve a loop of suture from within the eye. Cohesive viscoelastic in the anterior chamber will allow for the stable maintenance of space and easy removal at the end of the procedure.

Agarwal A, Agarwal A, eds. *Mastering Iris Repair: A Video Textbook of Iris Repair and Pupilloplasty Techniques* (pp 21-26).

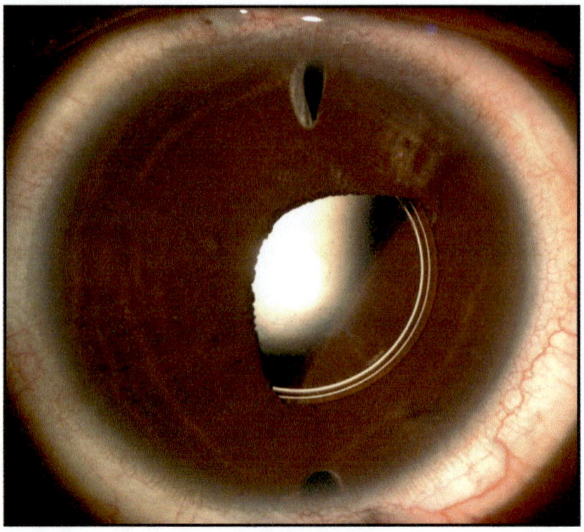

Figure 3-1. A case of optic capture after a glued IOL. This patient needs iris suturing. Note that despite 2 small iridectomies, an optic capture is still possible.

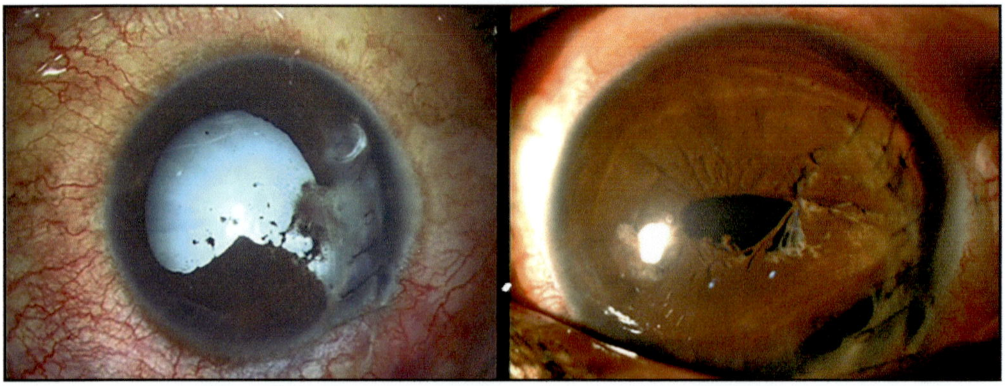

Figure 3-2. Preoperative and traumatic cataract with iris damage. This case featured an IOL implantation performed using the Siepser iris suturing technique.

Anesthesia

Expert surgeons can perform this maneuver using topical anesthesia with intracameral augmentation. For surgeons learning this technique, retrobulbar or peribulbar anesthesia may be preferred for better pain control.

Surgical Approach

The following is the recommended surgical approach for a simple radial tear in the iris sphincter. Other injuries or defects can be repaired using the Siepser technique, but surgeons should be comfortable with the steps of the procedure on simple iris repair prior to attempting more complex procedures. The surgeon should be seated so that sutures can easily be passed forehand or backhand, depending on surgeon preference. An initial 1-mm paracentesis incision should be made perpendicular to the iris defect at the nearest point parallel to the defect. For example, in the case of an inferior iris tear extending peripherally from the iris sphincter, most surgeons would elect to sit superiorly. A paracentesis directed perpendicular to the defect would then be placed at the 7 o'clock position to allow for a right hand, forehand needle pass across the defect. A miotic agent is often placed into the anterior chamber to allow for the iris to approximate the undilated state and the surgeon to line up the leaflets of the iris as accurately as possible (Figures 3-1 and 3-2).

Surgical Technique

A 1-mm paracentesis is created as described previously. After the installation of a miotic agent followed by a cohesive viscoelastic through the paracentesis, the long curved CIF-4 needle on a 10-0 polypropylene suture can be gently introduced via the paracentesis. The needle can be passed through the proximal iris leaflet, across the defect, and then through the distal iris leaflet. The needle can then be passed through the peripheral cornea at a point in a straight line from the paracentesis incision. Adequate suture should be pulled through the anterior chamber to allow the suture to double-back across the anterior chamber. At least 4 cm of suture tail should be allowed to remain outside of the paracentesis incision. At this point, the suture will be crossing the anterior chamber, entering through the 7 o'clock paracentesis incision, through the anterior surface of the proximal iris leaflet, across the iris defect, through the posterior surface of the distal iris leaflet, and then out through the peripheral cornea, all in a straight line across the bottom third of the anterior segment. During the needle passes through the iris leaflet, counter-traction on the iris with an intraocular forceps may be desirable to prevent stretching, tearing, or distortion of the iris. In this case, an inferior paracentesis should be, created and the intraocular microforceps can be used to hold the iris leaflet secure as the needle pass is made. Once both of the iris leaflets are engaged by the suture and the needle has exited out of the distal limbus, then a small instrument, such as a Kuglen hook, is now passed through the paracentesis and engaged with the suture filament beyond the distal iris leaflet. Pulling slowly and smoothly, this loop of suture is then externalized via the paracentesis. At this moment, the surgeon should carefully ensure that the loop of suture and the proximal strand of suture are not entangled within the eye or in the corneal wound. The proximal suture strand and the 2 strands of the suture loop will all pass through the paracentesis and should be properly aligned in a parallel fashion. The proximal suture tail is then passed into the suture loop from above and wrapped twice around the middle strand of the suture loop, with the suture passes advancing toward the paracentesis. The outside strand of the loop should pass through the paracentesis, across the anterior chamber, and exit directly through the edge of the cornea. Now the 2 suture tails can be gently pulled away from each other causing the initial 2-throw knot to gently slip into the eye and cinch together the 2 iris leaflets. Great care should be taken to ensure even tension on each suture tail to make sure that no undue traction is placed across the iris. Failure to exercise caution with equal tension may lead to tearing of the iris tissue or disinsertion of the iris root. Either injury can lead to excessive bleeding that may quickly degrade the surgeon's view and prevent continued repair of the iris defect. Once the initial 2-throw loop has been cinched gently yet securely to close the iris defect, then the sequence of retrieving a loop of the distal suture and ensuring the loop exits the paracentesis without tangling is repeated. At this time, a single throw of the free suture tail is done through the loop from the bottom of the loop. Once again gentle, even traction is placed across both suture tails, and the loop with the second suture throw is pulled into the eye, locking the knot upon gentle tightening. A second single-throw pass is accomplished in exactly the same manner to finally secure the knot within the eye. The intraocular scissors are now introduced through the paracentesis, and the suture tails are cut close to the knot. The cut tails are removed from the eye. In many cases, 2 or 3 interrupted sutures may be required to close a linear iris defect. Each suture is passed and tied in the same manner.

Variations of the Siepser Technique

One variation of the Siepser technique is the single-pass four-throw approach.[3] The needle is passed as described previously and the loop of suture retrieved. When the free end of the proximal suture tail is passed into the retrieved loop of suture, 4 throws are accomplished instead of 2. When the suture tails are gently tensioned the resulting knot creates a self-locking helical structure that does not require any further locking throws to secure the knot. This approach saves time and surgical maneuvers, but caution should be taken when tensioning the four-throw helix because more tension is required to secure the knot as it passes into the eye. Great care must be taken to ensure no traction is put on the iris or iris root when properly tensioning the 4-throw helix.

A second variation of the Siepser sliding knot is a series of passes that will result in the suture knot being inverted beneath the iris.[4] The advantage of this technique is that, with the knot buried beneath the iris, future endothelial keratoplasty will be easier because there will be a decreased chance of damage to the graft endothelium by the exposed knot in the anterior chamber. This approach is done with a paracentesis in both the proximal and distal limbus. As the needle is passed out of the distal paracentesis, it is docked into a cannula to avoid catching any corneal fibers. The needle is passed back across the anterior chamber twice to allow for the suture tails to exit the bottom of the iris instead of the anterior iris surface, thus ensuring that the resulting knot will ultimately be posterior to the iris.

The Siepser sliding knot technique is a valuable skill that allows for intraocular knot tying within the eye in a closed system while avoiding unnecessary intraocular maneuvers. Practice is critical to learn the proper steps and suture orientation. Preparation prior to surgery is necessary to allow for the smooth and successful execution of this technique.

Case Presentation

Cionni Technique for Iris Coloboma Repair

Robert J. Cionni, MD

A patient presented with a coloboma of the iris. The problem with using the standardized techniques for iris coloboma repair is that after the iris is repaired the pupil is decentered. To solve this issue, surgeons can bisect the iris sphincter tissue to separate the central iris sphincter from the peripheral one. This can be done using microscissors. Subsequently, the cut edges of the central sphincter can be sutured. The peripheral iris remnants are then stretched and sutured (Figure 3-3 and Video 3-3).

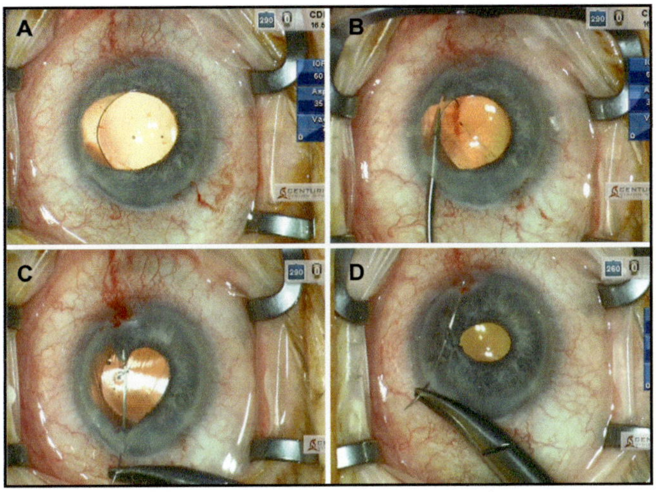

Figure 3-3. Cionni technique for iris coloboma repair. (A) Iris coloboma. (B) Central sphincter is cut with microscissors and separated from the peripheral iris. (C) Central iris is sutured. (D) Peripheral iris is then sutured.

References

1. Siepser SB. The closed chamber slipping suture technique for iris repair. *Ann Ophthalmol.* 1994;26(3):71-72.
2. Osher RH, Snyder ME, Cionni RJ. Modification of the Siepser slip-knot technique. *J Cataract Refract Surg.* 2005;31(6):1098-1100.
3. Narang P, Agarwal A. Single-pass four-throw technique for pupilloplasty. *Eur J Ophthalmol.* 2017;27:506-508.
4. Schoenberg ED, Price FW Jr. Modification of Siepser sliding suture technique for iris repair and endothelial keratoplasty. *J Cataract Refract Surg.* 2014;40(5):705-708.

Please visit www.routledge.com/9781630917265

to access additional material.

4

The Iris Cerclage Suture

Brandon D. Ayres, MD

Keywords

atonic pupil, iris cerclage, iris coloboma, iris defect, prosthetic lenses, pupilloplasty

The atonic, or permanently dilated, pupil can be a challenge for both patients and physicians. Patients will often complain of severe glare, photophobia, and haloing in almost all lighting conditions, indoors and out. For some patients, sunglasses will have to be worn at all times and the severe glare prevents them from enjoying everyday activities. Patients are not only bothered by light, but some are also bothered by the pupil's cosmetic appearance.[1,2]

Multiple causes for a dilated and nonreactive pupil have been reported. By far the most common etiology is ocular trauma. Less common causes can be viral infections, ocular surgery, neurologic conditions, angle-closure glaucoma, toxic anterior ischemic syndrome, diabetes, and Urrets-Zavalia syndrome. Treatment is indicated for symptomatic patients. In the majority of cases, pharmacologic agents will be ineffective. Tinted glasses and contact lenses can be effective for some patients. In cases with severe glare, an iris prosthesis contact lenses with a light-blocking background can be used. In some cases, patients who are unable to tolerate contact lenses will seek out surgical options.

Surgical correction for an iris defect includes techniques for iris repair or replacement. Several devices exist for iris replacement, including aniridic capsular tension rings, aniridic intraocular lenses (IOLs), and iris prosthesis (Figure 4-1). All of these devices will require removal of the cataract prior to placement. The capsular tension devices require an intact capsular bag for use. The silicone iris prosthesis and prosthetic IOL may be suture fixated if capsular support is not an option. Cost and access can also be problematic with these devices, as they are not approved for use in all areas. In some cases, the iris can be adequately repaired instead of replaced. Iris repair may

Agarwal A, Agarwal A, eds. *Mastering Iris Repair: A Video Textbook of Iris Repair and Pupilloplasty Techniques* (pp 27-34).

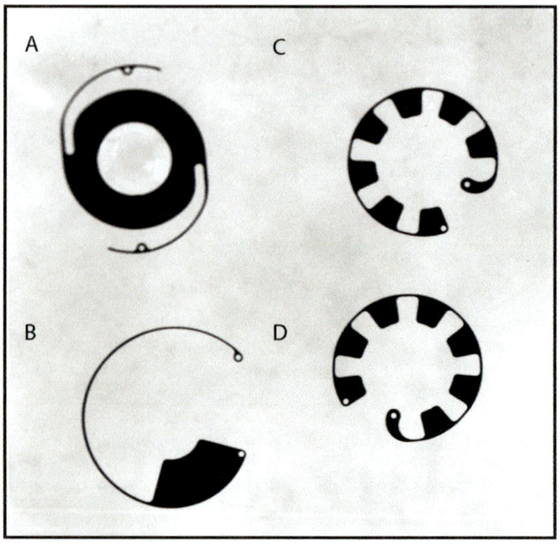

Figure 4-1. Three different devices for repair of iris defects. (A) A large polymethyl methacrylate aniridic implant. (B) A capsular tension ring with an iris segment to help patient with segmental iris defects. (C, D) Capsular tension ring with aniridic fins that compress when in the capsular bag creating an artificial iris aperture.

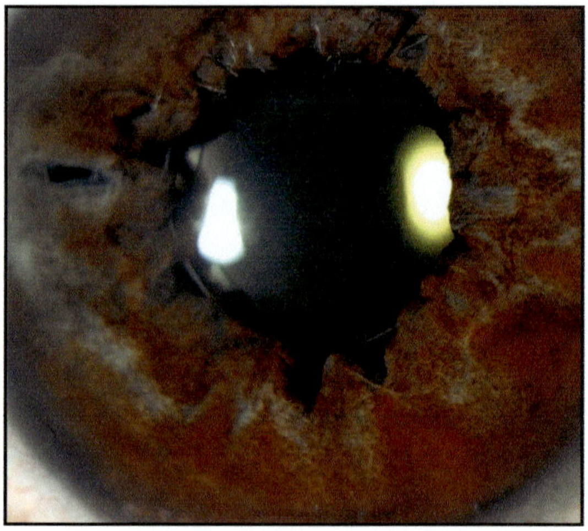

Figure 4-2. Iris cerclage.

be more economical than replacement and does not require implantation of a foreign body in the eye. In the correct clinical setting, an iris cerclage suture may be an excellent option for patients with an atonic pupil (Figure 4-2).[1]

Physical Examination

A complete ophthalmic examination is essential when evaluating a patient with a symptomatic iris defect. While all components of the slit-lamp examination are essential, it is important to highlight a few essential components. One critical part of the evaluation is examination of the unaffected eye in mesopic conditions to document pupil size so that it can be closely matched during surgery.

Evaluation of the corneal endothelial health is advisable. Many patients requiring iris repair have had ocular trauma and/or prior ocular surgical procedures. In some cases, cataract removal will also be necessary. A cell count will help inform the physician of the potential need for future corneal surgery and determine proper patient counseling. A detailed examination of the anterior chamber and iris, including gonioscopy, can give valuable information to the surgeon. Areas of peripheral anterior synechiae or posterior synechiae will need to be managed for a cerclage suture to be successful. Areas of severe pigment loss and iris stromal atrophy may be an indicator of iris elasticity, which can make iris repair difficult or even impossible.

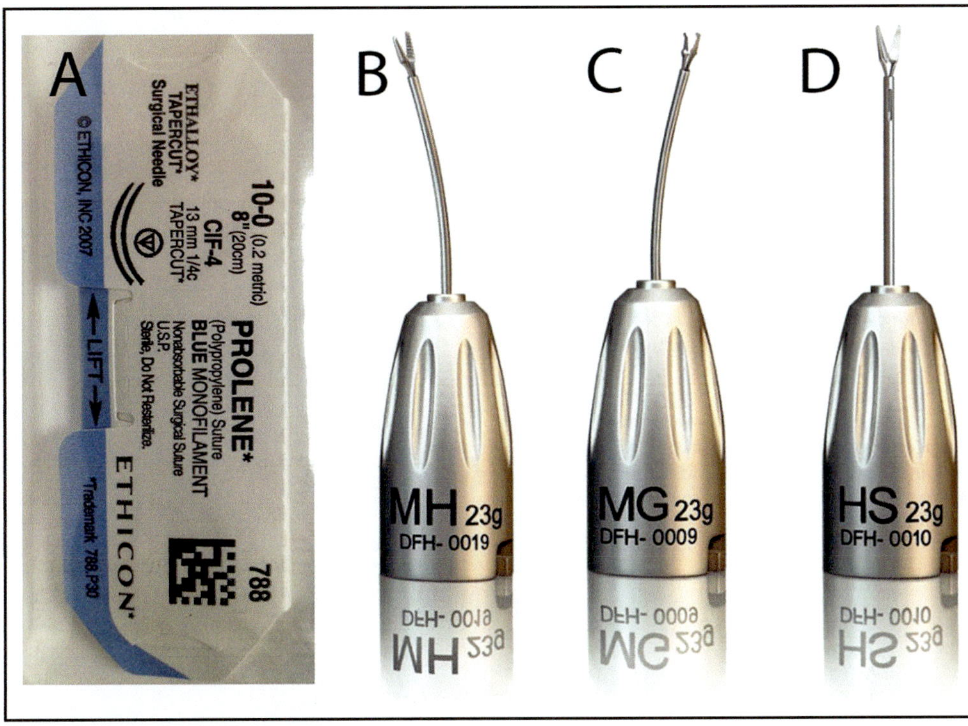

Figure 4-3. (A) 10-0 polypropylene suture on a long and curved tapercut needle used for iris suture. (B) Microforceps for use in the anterior chamber with a grasping jaw to prevent damage to iris tissue. (C) Microforceps with a downturned grasping jaw that can be helpful for holding iris tissue. (D) Intraocular scissors that can be used for cutting a suture in the anterior chamber.

The status of the lens or IOL should be noted, as well as any vitreous prolapse. A patient should not be left phakic with iris cerclage surgery. Cataract surgery before or at the time of the cerclage suture should be planned. If the patient is pseudophakic, it is critical to ensure that the IOL is stable. Biometry should be performed so that a backup IOL can be on hand in the operating room in the event that the current IOL dislocates during the procedure. If vitreous prolapse is present, it should be managed with anterior or posterior vitrectomy prior to placement of the suture.

A careful posterior segment examination should also be documented to make sure no retinal pathology needs treatment prior to closure of the pupil. It may also be advisable to speak with the retinal specialist to make sure the cerclage will not interfere with future retinal examinations or treatment.

Materials

Prior to tackling an iris cerclage suture, a few specialty devices will be necessary in the operating room. A 10-0 polypropylene suture will be needed for the cerclage. The polypropylene suture should be on a long, curved vascular needle, such as the CIF-4 (Ethicon). The vascular needle will not cut large holes in the delicate iris tissue as the suture is placed. Intraocular grasping forceps will also be necessary to manipulate the iris tissue. The forceps should be 23 to 25 gauge, curved, and with a broad grasping jaw. The curved shaft of the forceps will facilitate working in the anterior chamber, helping with the awkward maneuvers required by the cerclage suture. A pincher grasping forceps, such as internal limiting membrane forceps, should not be used for this technique because they may cause tears in the iris stroma (Figure 4-3). An ophthalmic viscosurgical device (OVD) will also be required for this procedure. The OVD will serve 2 purposes: it will help maintain the anterior chamber, and the OVD cannula will guide the 10-0 polypropylene needle out of the eye.

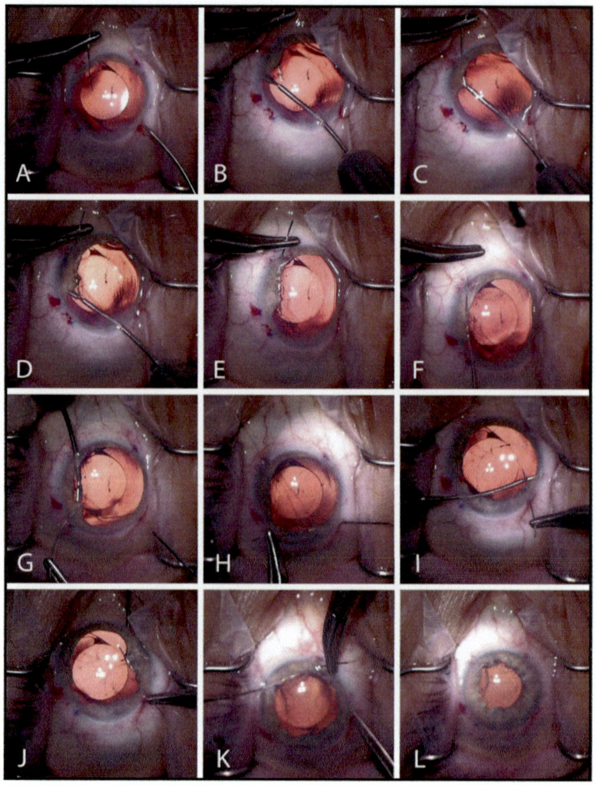

Figure 4-4. Surgical technique for iris cerclage suture. (A) A single-armed 10-0 polypropylene suture on a long, curved needle is placed through a paracentesis. (B) Using microforceps through a different paracentesis, the iris is grasped and stretched allowing the needle to pierce the iris near the pupil border. (C to E) The needle and microforceps are used to make a spiraling suture trying to capture 4 bites of the iris border prior to exiting through a paracentesis. (F) The OVD cannula is placed through the paracentesis, and the suture needle is docked into the lumen allowing it to safely exit the eye. (G, H) The needle is placed back into the paracentesis last exited and, using the microforceps, 4 additional spiraling iris bites are made before exiting the next paracentesis. (I, J) In a similar fashion, the needle is passed between 2 more paracenteses and then (K, L) brought around to the original incision used. Both ends of the suture are now extending through the same incision and are ready for tying.

Technique

Prior to placing the cerclage suture in the iris border, it is critical that all other anterior segment work be completed. The anterior chamber should be filled with OVD prior to placement of the suture. Four evenly spaced iris plane paracenteses should be placed. The grasping forceps can be placed through one of the paracentesis incisions to grasp the iris border and test the elasticity of the iris. Any peripheral anterior synechiae or posterior synechiae should be lysed at this time.

The 10-0 polypropylene needle should be carefully placed through one of the paracenteses (Video 4-1). The overall procedure will require running the suture from paracentesis to paracentesis in a clockwise or counterclockwise direction. The goal is to pass the needle through the iris border 4 times or more with each suture pass. Special care needs to be taken not to grasp any fibrils of the cornea while placing the needle into the eye (Figure 4-4).

After passing the needle into the first paracentesis, the grasping forceps are used through a second paracentesis to grasp and stretch the iris toward the needle. The needle is then pierced through the iris. The iris is re-grasped by the microforceps a few millimeters from the needle. In a spiraling motion, the needle is rotated around the pupil border and once again brought anterior to the iris. With the help of the microforceps, the needle is pierced through the iris again creating a spiraling baseball-like suture. The needle is slowly advanced toward the adjacent paracentesis, trying to pass the needle through the iris border 4 times, before exiting the eye.

After several bites are taken on the iris, the needle is pointed toward the internal aspect of the paracentesis to be exited. The OVD cannula can then be placed through the exiting paracentesis. The needle is then docked into the lumen of the OVD cannula and guided out of the eye. This technique prevents the needle from grabbing the fibers of the cornea as it exits the eye.

The needle is then re-grasped and carefully placed into the eye through the same paracentesis that was just exited. With the help of the microforceps, the needle is guided toward the next paracentesis taking 4 bites on the peripheral iris using the same spiraling suture technique. The needle exits the eye using the OVD cannula. This process is continued 2 more times until the needle exits the eye through the paracentesis used to start the procedure. At this point, the 10-0 polypropylene suture should be laced 360 degrees around the pupil border with the entry and exit suture through the same paracentesis. Pulling on the 2 ends of the suture should allow constriction of the pupil, and the suture should be free of any incarceration in the corneal wounds.

Tying the Knot

The knot used to tie the cerclage suture is a modification of the McCannel technique. It is a 3 × 1 × 1 surgeon's knot tied outside the eye and then adjusted with one instrument outside the eye and a second inside the eye (Figure 4-5). After the cerclage suture is placed, both ends of the suture will be protruding through the same paracentesis incision. The triple throw portion of the surgeon's knot is made and tightened until the elasticity of the iris pulls the triple throw into the eye. To adjust the size of the pupil, one free end of the suture is grasped outside the eye with a tying forceps, and the other free end is grasped inside the eye with intraocular forceps and slowly adjusted by adding tension. Once the iris reaches the desired size, the suture is released. The 2 additional throws of the surgeon's knot can then be created. Each throw is started outside the eye and then drawn inward and tightened in a similar fashion to the initial 3 throws. After the knot is completed, the ends can be cut with intraocular scissors or a blade. The main advantages of this knot tying technique are excellent control of the pupil size and no excessive stress on the iris tissue.

Final Steps

After the cerclage suture is in place and tied, the last step is to remove the OVD from the anterior chamber. If the iris cerclage was the primary procedure, a bimanual irrigation aspiration unit can be used as it will not require a large incision. If a larger incision was made for cataract or an IOL, then a more traditional coaxial irrigation aspiration unit can be used. The procedure is complete after all incisions are sealed and Seidel negative.

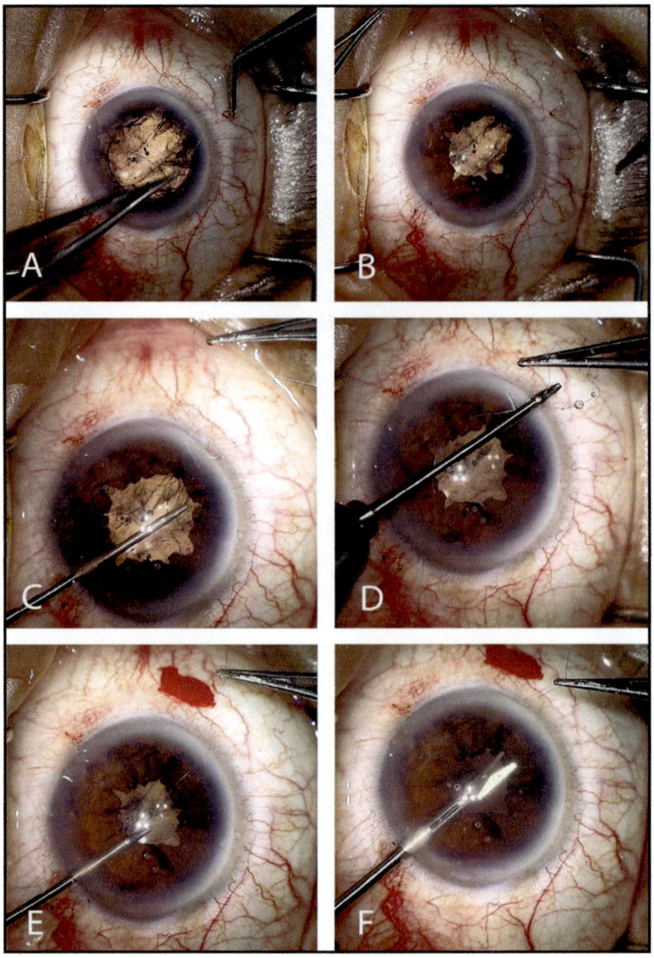

Figure 4-5. Tying the cerclage suture. (A) Starting with both ends of the suture extending through the same incision, the first 3 throws of a 3×1×1 surgeon's knot is started. (B) The suture is gently tightened, allowing the knot to drop into the anterior chamber. (C) With one end of the suture held outside the eye and the other end of the suture grasped in the anterior chamber, the tension is adjusted until the pupil is at the desired size. (D) Outside the eye, the second throw of the 3×1×1 surgeon's knot is made and allowed to prolapse into the anterior chamber. (E) One end of the suture is grasped outside the eye and other end is grasped with microforceps and tightened, thus locking the suture. This process is repeated one more time completing the 3×1×1 surgeon's knot. (F) Once complete, the suture ends are cut in the anterior chamber using microscissors.

Case Presentation

Subluxated Intraocular Lens in a Large Eye With Iris Cerclage

Priya Narang, MS; Ashvin Agarwal, MBBS, MS; and Amar Agarwal, MS, FRCS, FRCOphth

A subluxated IOL in a large eye was refixed using the glued IOL technique. The patient also had a mydriasis so an iris cerclage was performed. In this procedure, the Prolene (Ethicon) needle with suture is passed around the pupil so that an entire cerclage is completed (Figure 4-6 and Video 4-2).

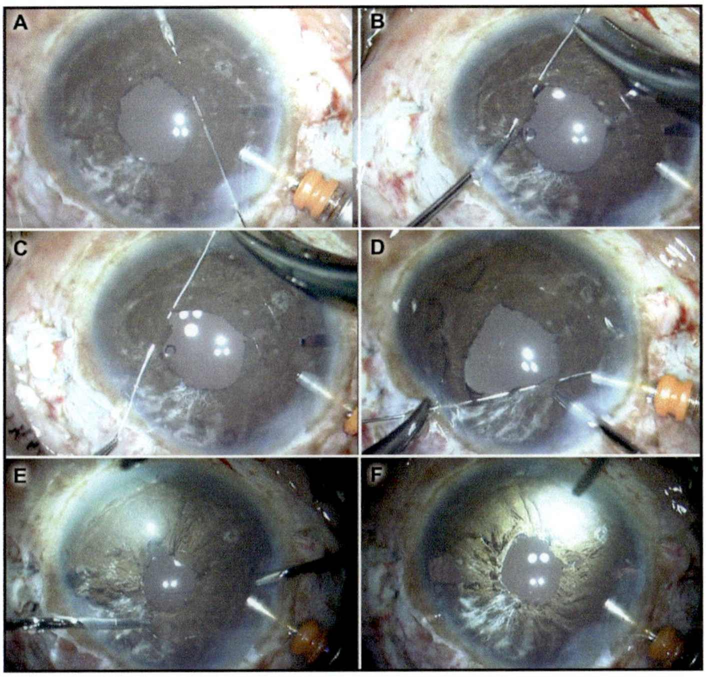

Figure 4-6. Iris cerclage. (A) The Prolene suture with needle is passed through small bites of the iris and brought out through the opposite clear corneal opening. (B) The second quadrant is done. (C) The needle is brought out again through a clear corneal wound. (D) The needle is once more passed into the anterior chamber and small bites of the iris are taken. (E) The suture is then tied. (F) A postoperative picture shows a successful iris cerclage.

References

1. Ogawa GS. The iris cerclage suture for permanent mydriasis: a running suture technique. *Ophthalmic Surg Lasers.* 1998;29(12):1001-1009.
2. McCannel MA. A retrievable suture idea for anterior uveal problems. *Ophthalmic Surg.* 1976;7(2):98-103.

Please visit www.routledge.com/9781630917265 to access additional material.

5

Mastering the Single-Pass Four-Throw Pupilloplasty

Priya Narang, MS; Ashvin Agarwal, MBBS, MS; Ashar Agarwal, MS, FRCS; and Amar Agarwal, MS, FRCS, FRCOphth

Keywords

corectopia, McCannel, pupil reconstruction, Siepser technique, single-pass four-throw pupilloplasty

Pupil reconstruction is an essential aspect to prevent photophobia and filter the amount of light that is needed in cases with traumatic mydriasis and atonic pupils. Surgical repair is of substantial benefit as it has the potential to reduce visual glare and light sensitivity. Amongst various techniques[1-9] that have been described for pupil reconstruction, single-pass four-throw (SFT) is one of the newer techniques that can be employed for pupilloplasty.[10] As the name suggests, a single pass of the Prolene (Ethicon) 10-0 suture on a long-armed needle is passed through the iris tissue followed by the creation of a loop with 4 throws around it that slides inside the eye like a Siepser sliding knot technique. This creates a helical configuration that prevents the suture from opening up (Figures 5-1 through 5-3). The SFT pupilloplasty technique involves a single pass in the anterior chamber followed by 4 throws taken through the loop that is withdrawn from the anterior chamber. The procedure has an approximation loop with no additional securing loop. Hence the traditional knot formation that involves multiple passes through the anterior chamber does not happen with the SFT procedure. The helical configuration created by intertwining the loop has a self-locking and self-retaining mechanism (Video 5-1).

Agarwal A, Agarwal A, eds. *Mastering Iris Repair: A Video Textbook of Iris Repair and Pupilloplasty Techniques* (pp 35-46).

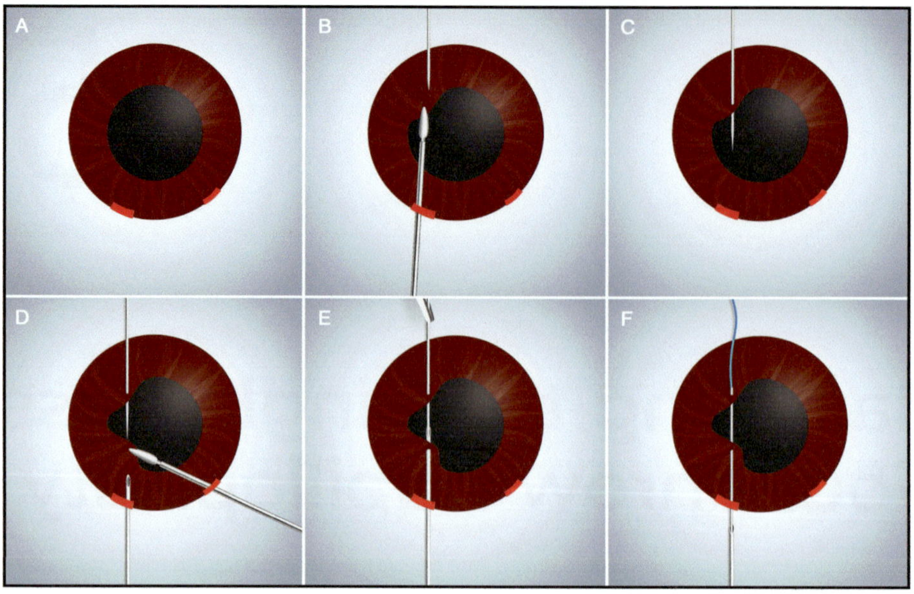

Figure 5-1. Illustration of SFT pupilloplasty. (A) Two paracentesis incisions serve as the site for introduction of an end-opening forceps and 26-gauge needle for performing pupilloplasty (paracentesis sites marked in red). (B) A 10-0 suture attached to the long arm of the needle is passed through the clear cornea. An end-opening forceps is introduced from the opposite end and the proximal part of the iris tissue that is to be repaired is held with the forceps. This makes the iris taut and facilitates its passage through the iris. (C) The 10-0 needle is passed through the proximal iris tissue. (D) A 26-gauge needle is introduced from the opposite side through the paracentesis incision and the iris edge is grasped by end-opening forceps introduced from the adjacent paracentesis incision. (E) The 10-0 needle is docked into the barrel of the 26-gauge needle. (F) The 10-0 needle is pulled and withdrawn from the anterior chamber through the paracentesis incision.

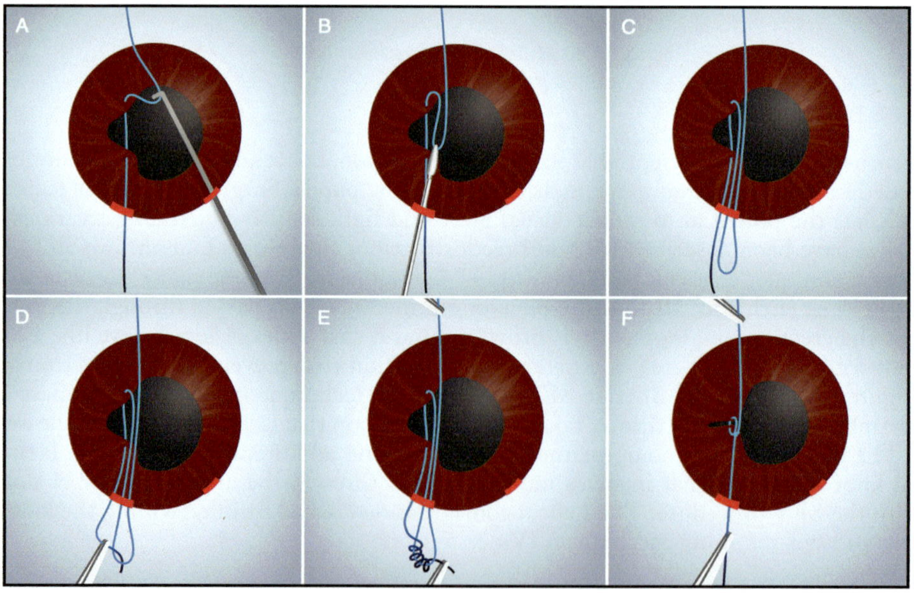

Figure 5-2. Illustration of SFT pupilloplasty. (A) Using a dialer, form a loop of the distal suture end intraocularly. (B) Using micrograspers/intraocular end-opening forceps externalize the loop via the paracentesis. (C) The distal suture loop is externalized through the paracentesis and maintained immediately outside the paracentesis. (D) The leading end of the suture is passed through the loop. (E) Four throws of the leading end are passed through the loop with care being taken to pass the suture through the loop in the same direction. (F) Pull both the distal and proximal end of the suture, internalizing the helical knot.

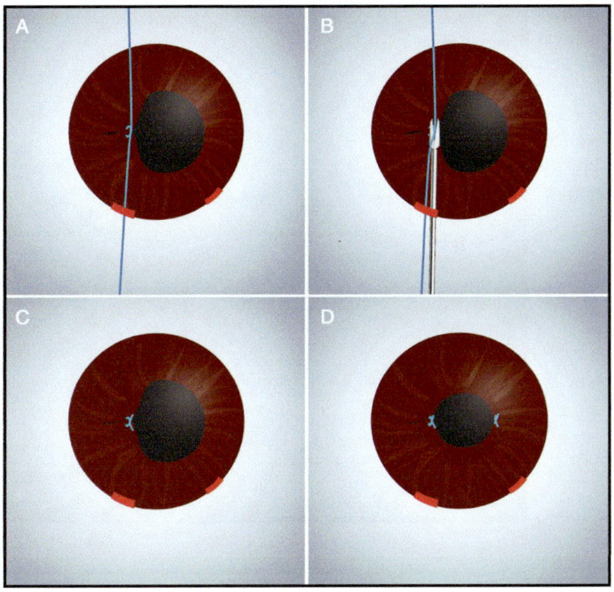

Figure 5-3. Illustration of SFT pupilloplasty. (A) Helical knot is formed. (B) Microscissors are used to cut the ends of the knot. (C) Pupilloplasty is complete on one side. (D) Pupilloplasty is complete on the other side with resultant desired pupil.

Knot Mechanics

Ashley's book of knots[11] describes various knot formation techniques that help hold an object together in weightbearing, as well as non-weightbearing, conditions. The method of helical knot formation of SFT has been described as a timber hitch (Figure 5-4), which is a common method employed in various outdoor activities and was described as early as 1762. Ashley's book[11] explains various types of knot formations including both the slip knot and timber hitch. The differences between the knots are minute, with knot formation changing with the addition or omission of a twist or a loop (Figure 5-5).

Mathematical analysis has been done to explain what causes a hitch to hold or loosen up.[12,13] Friction prevents the knot from slipping. Friction occurs when there is pressure at a place within the knot, which is called the *nip*.[11] In the SFT knot, friction occurs between the iris tissue and the suture thereby holding the knot in place (Figure 5-6).

If T2 is the force exerted toward the center and T1 is the force that acts to pull the iris tissue toward periphery, then the SFT loop will hold if $T2 > T1$. With 4 throws, $T2 > T1$ so the SFT loop holds. With less than 4 throws, the SFT loop loosens and opens up because $T2 < T1$. With the increase in throws, theoretically, more friction is created and more energy is needed to approximate and slide the loop internally. Four throws are optimal in preventing opening of the loop and creating a self-locking system, which happens to correlate with the timber hitch method.

The slippage of a hitch/knot can be mitigated by leaving plenty of rope at the working end of the knot, and by tightening it as much as possible before loading. Similarly, in SFT, before the suture ends are cut, pulling both suture ends ensures tightening of the loop across the iris tissue. Around 1 mm of suture end is left on either side to prevent slippage of the cut end inside the loop, which prevents it from loosening and eventually opening up. To the best of our knowledge, opening of the SFT loop has not been reported in any case when optimal 4 throws are taken in situ.

The indications of SFT are vast. They range from cases with traumatic mydriasis to optic capture and Urrets-Zavalia syndrome;[14] cases undergoing endothelial keratoplasty;[15] and in certain select cases of angle-closure glaucoma (ACG) with peripheral anterior synechiae.[16]

The following section briefly summarizes the indications for pupilloplasty.

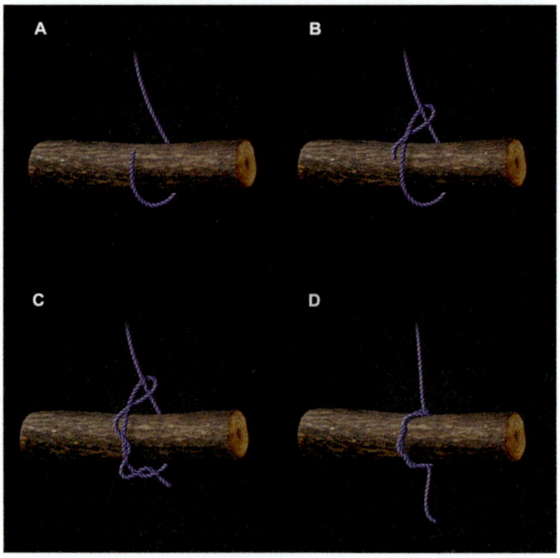

Figure 5-4. Illustration of the timber hitch. Illustration depicts the loop formation on a log of wood. (A) A rope is passed around the log. (B) One end of the rope is crossed over itself and a loop is created. (C) The rope is further tucked under itself and is looped around. (D) The rope end is pulled and the hitch engulfs the log circumference. (Reprinted with permission from Narang P, Agarwal A. Single-pass four-throw pupilloplasty knot mechanics. *J Refract Surg*. 2019;35[3]:207-208.)

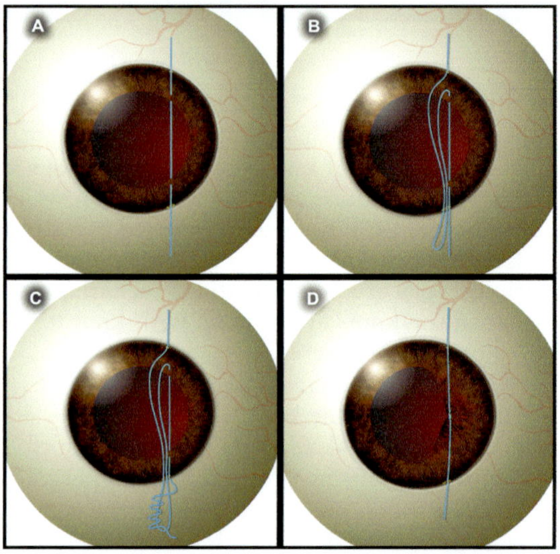

Figure 5-5. Illustration of SFT pupilloplasty comparison with timber hitch knot. (A) Needle passed through the proximal and distal portion of the iris tissue. (B) A loop of suture is withdrawn after approximation of the proximal and distal portion of the iris tissue. (C) The suture end is passed through the loop. This is similar to the clinical stage depicted in Figures 5-4A through 5-4C. (D) The suture ends are pulled and the loop slides inside approximating and holding the iris tissue. This simulates Figure 5-4D. (Reprinted with permission from Narang P, Agarwal A. Single-pass four-throw pupilloplasty knot mechanics. *J Refract Surg*. 2019;35[3]:207-208.)

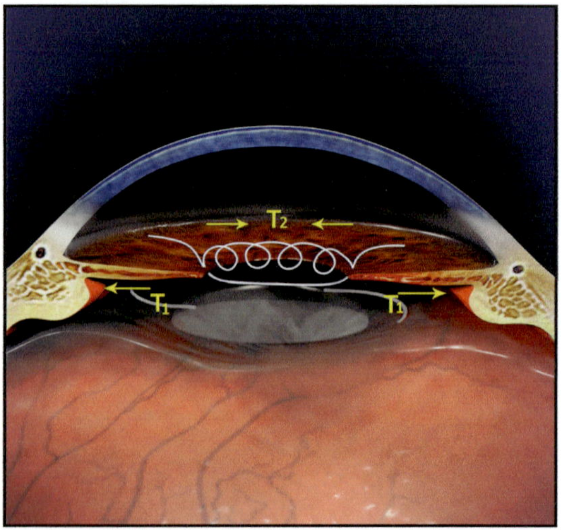

Figure 5-6. Mechanics of SFT pupilloplasty. The image depicts T2 and T1 forces exerted on the iris tissue. T2 is the frictional force that acts toward the center of the pupil, and T1 is the force exerted by the peripheral iris tissue. With 4 throws, T2 > T1, so SFT loops hold their position. With less than 4 throws, T2 < T1, so SFT loops open up. (Reprinted with permission from Narang P, Agarwal A. Single-pass four-throw pupilloplasty knot mechanics. *J Refract Surg*. 2019;35[3]:207-208.)

Indications

Pupilloplasty is indicated in the following conditions in symptomatic patients:

- Corneal indications
  - Endothelial keratoplasty like pre-Descemet's endothelial keratoplasty (especially in aphakic eyes or those with a deficient posterior capsule, so as to prevent the graft from getting displaced in the posterior segment and to maintain an adequate anterior chamber for graft unrolling and placement)
- Glaucoma related
  - ACG
  - Plateau iris syndrome
  - Broad peripheral anterior synechiae
- Pupil-related indications
  - Traumatic mydriasis
  - Urrets-Zavalia syndrome
  - Iatrogenic iridectomies
  - Iris defect (eg, congenital coloboma iris, corectopia, polycoria)
- Intraocular lens (IOL)–related indications
  - Optic capture
  - Glued IOL
  - Prevention of posterior synechiae

Relative Contraindications

- Phakic eyes with clear lens
- Atrophic iris

Surgical Technique

The amount of iris defect should be initially assessed, and an imaginary line drawn from the intended edges of the defect to the limbus. This marks the paracentesis site. Another paracentesis should be made approximately 45 to 90 degrees away (see Figure 5-1A). In cases with traumatic mydriasis, Urrets-Zavalia syndrome, ACG, pupillary stretching is performed with end-opening forceps to pull the iris on every clock hour and break any possible synechiae that might be present. This step also helps give the immobile iris some elasticity (see Figures 5-1 through 5-3).

It is a good practice to begin such surgeries with an anterior chamber maintainer (ACM) or a trocar anterior chamber maintainer (TACM)[17] with infusion of fluid in the eye (Video 5-2). Alternatively, the surgeon can perform the procedure with viscoelastic (if posterior capsule is intact) in the anterior chamber. The viscoelastic should be meticulously washed out from within the anterior chamber to avoid any inflammation or intraocular pressure spike postoperatively. In the case of glued IOL, aphakic patients, or those with a deficient posterior capsule, the use of viscoelastic is not recommended because of the possibility of viscoelastic entering the posterior segment. In such cases, an ACM or a TACM can be used with infusion of balanced salt solution in the eye.

With an end-opening forceps introduced through the paracentesis, grasp one edge of the iris defect (see Figure 5-1B). With the other hand, enter the eye using a 9-0 or 10-0 Prolene suture on a straight, long needle through the clear cornea and through the iris. At this time, the needle can be released (see Figure 5-1C). Introduce an end-opening forceps through the other paracentesis and grasp the other edge of the iris defect. Pass a 26-gauge needle through the primary paracentesis, and then pass it through the iris. The surgeon can now release the iris, railroad the Prolene suture into the needle and externalize the 10-0 suture needle (see Figures 5-1D through 5-1F). At this time, the intraocular Prolene suture can be divided into 3 parts: the distal, intermediate, and proximal. Using a dialer or a Sinskey hook, engage the distal part of the suture and form a loop in the anterior chamber (see Figure 5-2A). Externalize this loop using micrograspers, taking care to maintain the externalized loop immediately outside the paracentesis (see Figures 5-2B and 5-2C). At this stage, it is important to ensure that neither of the suture parts has crossed over each other.

The leading end of the suture can now be cut. This end is passed into the loop of the suture 4 times (see Figures 5-2D and 5-2E). This entails the 4 throws of the SFT technique. Once this is done, pull on both ends of the suture (see Figure 5-2F). The helical knot that is thus formed slides into the eye and the pupil approximation is achieved (see Figure 5-3A). The microscissors are employed to cut the ends of the suture making sure the suture ends are neither too short nor too long (see Figure 5-3B and 5-3C). The SFT procedure (see Video 5-1) is then repeated in the other quadrant to achieve the suitable and required size of the pupil (see Figure 5-3D).

Complications

- Cataract: When pupilloplasty is done in a phakic patient, the chances of lens touch and subsequent cataract formation is high. To avoid this possible complication, combine cataract extraction with IOL implantation in the bag and then proceed with SFT.
- Intraocular hemorrhage: Hyphema rarely occurs with the procedure. This is usually self-limiting and resolves spontaneously over a period of 1 to 2 weeks.
- Iatrogenic iris trauma: This may occur, especially in cases where atrophic iris is preexistent.
- Iridodialysis: This occurs when the bites that are taken are too large, and involves a large area of the iris tissue. In such cases, tying of the suture knot causes traction on the peripheral iris that can induce iatrogenic iridodialysis.
- Endothelial damage due to inadvertent touch of the endothelium with the suture needle.
- Suture passing through the corneal tissue rather than the paracentesis. To avoid this, pass the 26-gauge needle in a rocking fashion through the paracentesis so that the needle does not go through the corneal tissue.

Advantages

- Simple, straightforward procedure that is less time consuming.
- Because only a single pass is needed through the iris, there is minimal iris manipulation and, therefore, the possibility of iris tissue damage and inflammatory reaction due to iris pigment release is minimized.
- Pupillary dilatation is possible even after 2 or 3 SFTs have been performed in an eye, because there is enough viable iris tissue and the elasticity of the pupil is maintained.[18] It has been found that a pupil can be dilated to about 3 times its area even after SFT (eg, a postoperative SFT pupil the size of 5 mm^2 can be dilated to 13 mm^2 with regular dilatation). Therefore, this procedure is ideal for cases with potential or existing retinal disease (Figure 5-7).

Discussion

SFT pupilloplasty is a simple procedure that has varied applications and several advantages (Figures 5-8 and 5-9). The most important advantage of performing SFT is that the pupil has been documented to dilate after instillation of mydriatics, which was quantified on anterior segment optical coherence tomography analysis. Post-mydriatic instillation, a clinically significant increase in pupillary size occurred with higher mydriasis in the vertical axis as compared to the horizontal axis. The induced mydriasis was significant and is conceptualized to aid in fundus visualization and monitoring of glaucoma progression. In patients with a preoperatively high intraocular pressure and closed angles, SFT now acts as a mechanical miotic holding the iris tight and in position, thus preventing the iris from ever occluding the angles again. In patients with preoperative glare and halos, the amount of light entering the eye is restricted and the pupil is given a more physiological size, hence the patient is relieved of his or her symptoms. As such, there are no absolute contraindications to SFT (Figure 5-10 and Video 5-3). Relative contraindication being a phakic eye with a clear lens due to the possibility of lens touch and cataract formation,

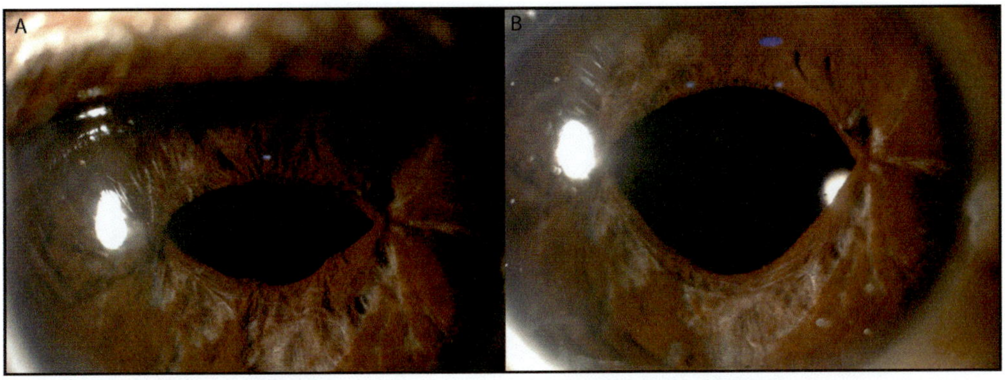

Figure 5-7. Dilatation of the pupil after SFT. (A) Pre-dilation pupil after SFT and (B) 40 minutes after dilation with Tropicacyl (tropicamide). (Reprinted with permission from Chang DF, ed. *Advanced IOL Fixation Techniques: Strategies for Compromised or Missing Capsular Support*. Thorofare, NJ: SLACK Incorporated; 2019.)

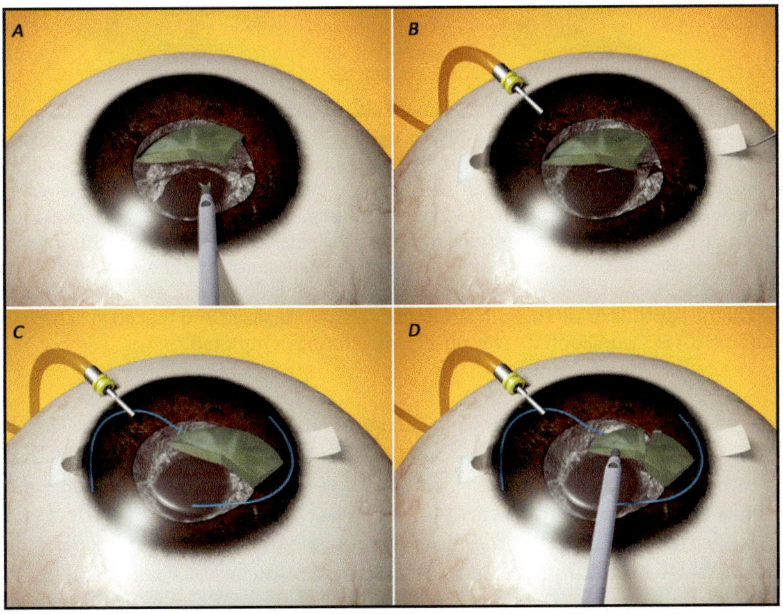

Figure 5-8. Part 1: SFT pupilloplasty used in triumvirate technique for sinking nucleus in deficient capsule support. (A) Posterior capsule rupture with sinking nucleus. (B) Two partial-thickness scleral flaps made 180 degrees opposite to each other. The TACM is introduced at a distance of 0.5 mm away from the limbus creating bi-planar incision architecture. Scleral flap lifted and sclerotomy being made with 22-gauge needles approximately 1.5 mm away from the limbus. A rod being introduced from the sclerotomy incision for performing posterior assisted levitation. The rod is positioned and placed beneath the nuclear fragments to levitate it in anterior chamber. (C) Nucleus lying in anterior chamber. A 3-piece foldable IOL is inserted beneath the nuclear fragments into the anterior chamber in a way that it blocks the pupillary area and the IOL rests on the anterior surface of the iris. (D) Phaco probe introduced into the anterior chamber and IOL scaffold procedure being performed with moderate parameters.

and an atrophic iris due to the possibility of an iridodialysis and increased iris damage. SFT can be performed in patients with clear lens in conjunction with a lens extraction and IOL placement in the bag because lens extraction is currently deemed as one of the surgical maneuvers in patients with ACG.

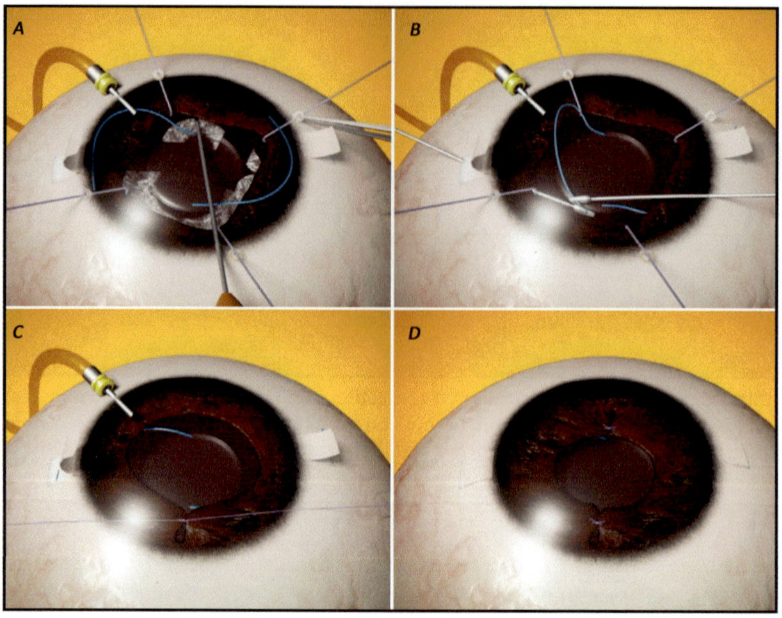

Figure 5-9. Part 2: SFT pupilloplasty used in triumvirate technique for sinking nucleus in deficient capsule support. (A) Entire nucleus emulsified and retropupillary cortex visualized. The corneal wound is sutured and vitrectomy is performed with a 23-gauge probe inserted from the sclerotomy site. Thorough cortical removal with adequate vitrectomy is performed. The entire IOL rests on the iris tissue in the anterior chamber. (B) Glued IOL forceps introduced from the sclerotomy site and a side-port incision holds the haptic of the IOL. Handshake technique being performed until the tip of the haptic is grasped. Both the haptics are externalized and tucked in Scharioth pocket. (C) SFT pupilloplasty started. (D) Iris suturing completed.

In conclusion, SFT adds to our arsenal as surgeons in a vast majority of cases. From repairing closed angles to avoiding the debilitating effects of an optic capture and normalizing pupil size, the SFT procedure works in many ways. We advocate the use of SFT in cases of Urrets-Zavalia syndrome to avoid the possible complications of contact lenses and to provide a permanent treatment option. The learning curve for this procedure is short and is easy to replicate. Surgeons can aptly learn and apply this technique to help as many patients as they can.

Trocar Anterior Chamber Maintainer

Maintenance of a deep anterior chamber is a prerequisite for a safe, smooth intraocular surgery as it prevents inadvertent and harmful touch to the corneal endothelium. It is for this reason that a viscoelastic device was introduced. It served as a major breakthrough for all anterior segment intraocular surgeries. The ACM has to be introduced via a corneal paracentesis incision using a side port or a microvitreoretinal blade. An incision that is too large can often cause the ACM to be expelled from the eye, and an incision that is too small necessitates further enlargement that may or may not be the exact dimension. We introduced an improvised TACM technique used in posterior segment surgeries. The TACM (see Video 5-2) is inserted into the anterior chamber from the limbus to maintain adequate infusion into the eye during the surgical maneuver. This is made by Mastel.

TACM is a 25-gauge stainless needle and cannula. It has an inner trocar needle that slides directly through the cornea leaving the cannula in place (Figure 5-11). The TACM comes as a surgical package of a trocar needle with cannula with handle, the protective cover, and the infusion tube line (Figure 5-12). A distance of 0.5 mm from the limbus is measured and marked using a vernier caliper and then the trocar is introduced at a 45-degree angle to the sclera, parallel to the limbus by displacing the conjunctiva. The trocar is then turned 90 degrees perpendicular to the

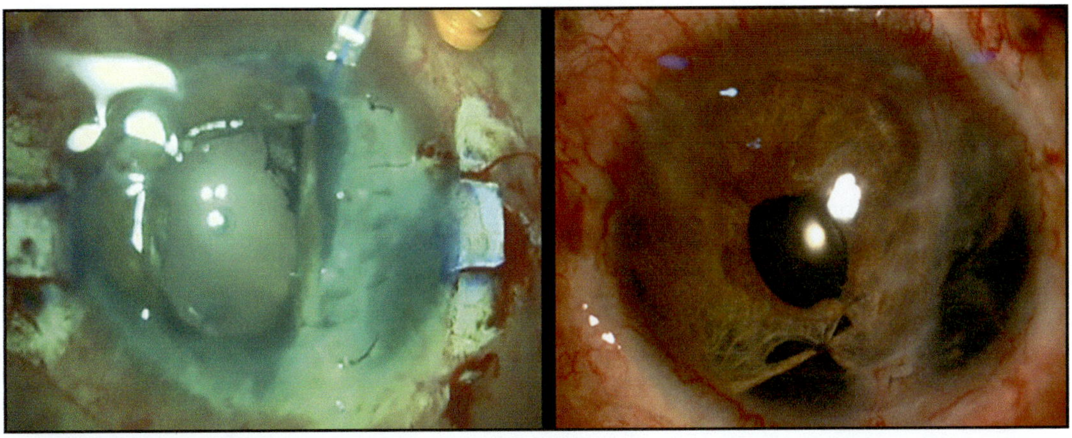

Figure 5-10. Pre- and postoperative traumatic case of glued IOL with SFT.

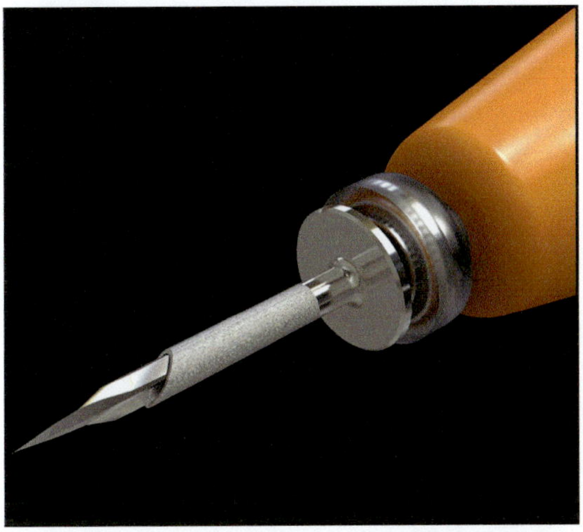

Figure 5-11. TACM surgical package set contains the trocar needle with cannula, protective cover, and infusion tube line.

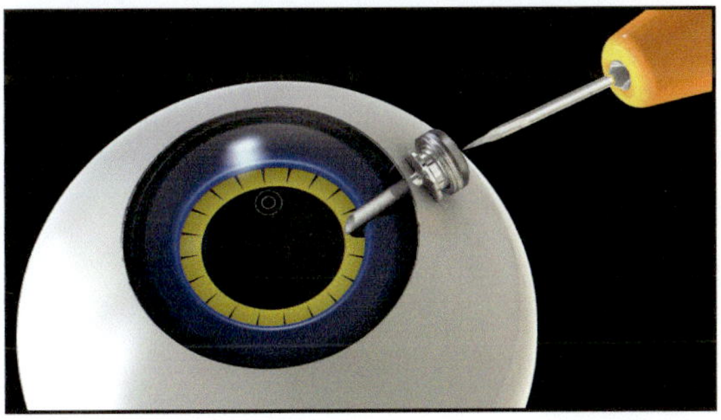

Figure 5-12. Illustration showing the insertion of TACM.

limbus and directed toward the anterior chamber so the trocar enters the anterior chamber in front of the iris tissue. The cannula is flushed to the surface of the sclera, and the trocar is withdrawn, leaving the cannula in place. The infusion line is then attached to the hub of the cannula and the infusion turned on. One can alternatively make a straight entry into the sclera above the iris.

We suggest always using a TACM in cases of iris repair rather than using viscoelastic alone. This makes using a vitrectomy probe to adjust the size of the pupil easy as fluid is always in the eye, and any iris bleeding gets washed away by the fluid.

Case Presentation 1

Single-Pass Four-Throw Pupilloplasty

Priya Narang, MS and Amar Agarwal, MS, FRCS, FRCOphth

A young male presented with a history of trauma associated with dimness of vision in his right eye. Slit-lamp examination revealed a subluxated cataract with traumatic mydriasis. Secondary IOL implantation with glued intrascleral technique was planned for the case after removal of cataractous lens. SFT technique was performed to correct the traumatic mydriasis (Figure 5-13 and Video 5-4).

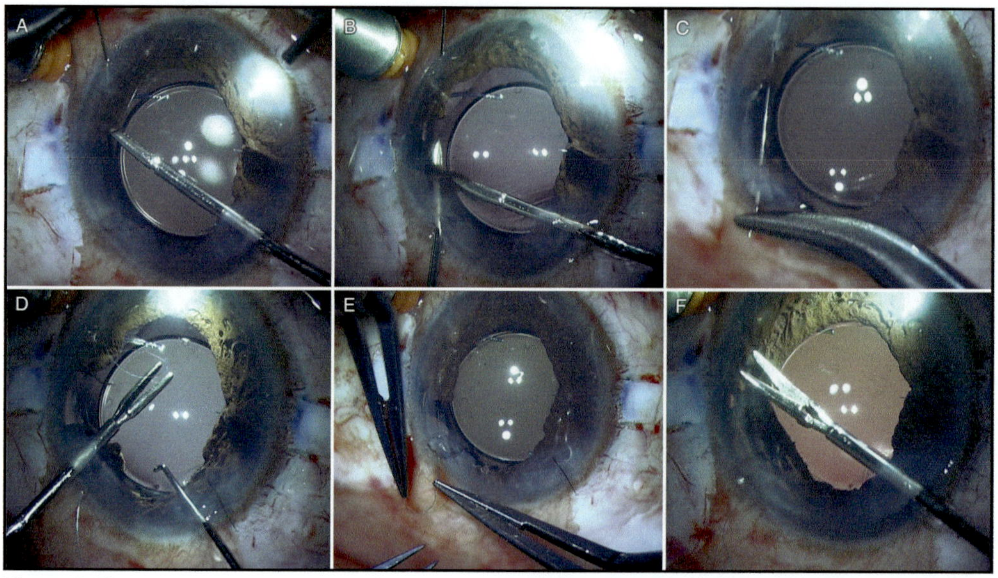

Figure 5-13. SFT pupilloplasty surgical technique. (A) The proximal end of the iris leaflet is held with an end-opening forceps and a 10-0 long-armed needle is passed through it from the side port incision. (B) A 26-gauge needle is passed through the opposite side from the distal edge of the iris tissue. (C) The long-armed needle is passed into the barrel of the 26-gauge needle and pulled out of the eye. (D) A Sinskey hook is passed, and it engages the suture that is pulled inside the anterior chamber, creating a loop. (E) The loop is pulled out and the suture end is passed 4 times through the loop. (F) Both ends of the suture are pulled and this leads to the sliding of the loops inside the anterior chamber. After the loops are secured the suture is cut in a way that it leaves 1 mm of end on either side.

Case Presentation 2

Yamane Technique With Single-Pass Four-Throw Pupilloplasty

Sadeer B. Hannush, MD

A patient presented with aphakia and iris defects. In such a case, one has to implant an IOL and at the same time solve the iris defect. An intrascleral haptic fixation with the Yamane technique was done. This was followed by a SFT pupilloplasty surgery to solve the iris defect (Figure 5-14 and Video 5-5).

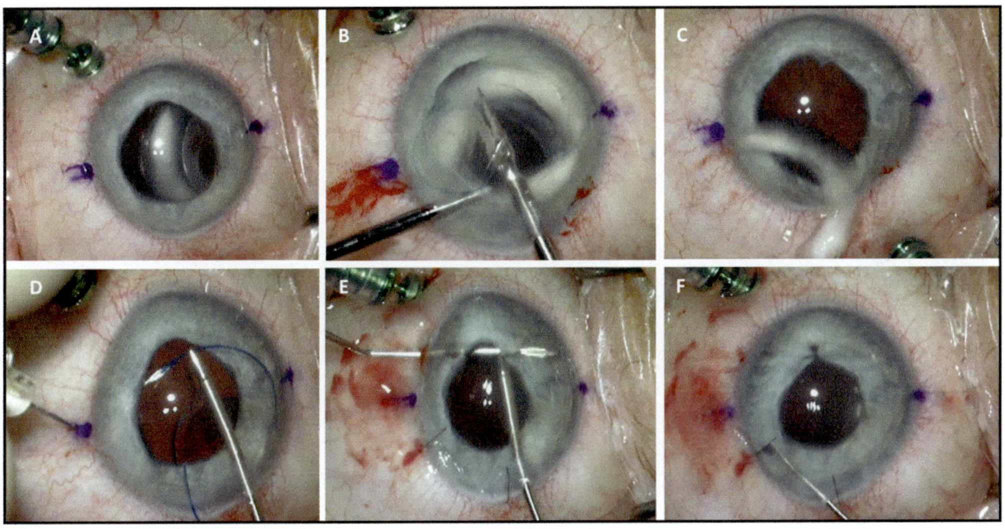

Figure 5-14. Yamane technique with SFT pupilloplasty. (A) Subluxated capsular bag intraocular complex. (B) The IOL is cut and explanted. (C) The Soemmering rings are removed. (D) Yamane technique performed. (E) SFT pupilloplasty is started. (F) SFT pupilloplasty is completed.

References

1. Siepser SB. The closed-chamber slipping suture technique for iris repair. *Ann Ophthalmol.* 1994;26:71-72.
2. Osher RH, Snyder ME, Cionni RJ. Modification of the Siepser slip-knot technique. *J Cataract Refract Surg.* 2005;31:1098-1100.
3. Snyder ME, Osher RH. Techniques and principles of surgical management of the traumatic cataract. In: Steinert RF, ed. *Cataract Surgery: Techniques, Complications and Management*, 2nd ed. Philadelphia, PA: Saunders; 2004;331-329.
4. Chang DF. Siepser slipknot for McCannel iris-suture fixation of subluxated intraocular lenses. *J Cataract Refract Surg.* 2004;30:1170-1176.
5. McCannel MA. A retrievable suture idea for anterior uveal problems. *Ophthalmic Surg.* 1976;7:98-103.
6. Ogawa GSH. The iris cerclage suture for permanent mydriasis: a running suture technique. *Ophthalmic Surg Lasers.* 1998;29:1001-1009.
7. Wachler BS, Krueger RR. Double-armed McCannel suture for repair of traumatic iridodialysis. *Am J Ophthalmol.* 1996;122:109-110.
8. Kaufman SC, Insler MS. Surgical repair of a traumatic iridodialysis. *Ophthalmic Surg Lasers.* 1996;27:963-966.
9. Schoenberg ED, Price FW Jr. Modification of Siepser sliding suture technique for iris repair and endothelial keratoplasty. *J Cataract Refract Surg.* 2014;40:705-708.
10. Narang P, Agarwal A. Single-pass four-throw technique for pupilloplasty. *Eur J Ophthalmol.* 2017;27:506-508.
11. Ashley CW. *The Ashley Book of Knots.* New York, NY: Doubleday; 1944;12.
12. Bayman BF. Theory of hitches. *Amer J Phys.* 1977:45;185-190.
13. Maddocks JH, Keller JB. Ropes in equilibrium. *SIAM J Appl Math.* 47;1987:1185-1200.
14. Narang P, Agarwal A. Single pass four-throw pupilloplasty for Urrets-Zavalia syndrome. *Eur J Ophthalmol.* 2018;28(5):552-558. doi: 10.1177/1120672117747038
15. Narang P, Agarwal A, Kumar DA. Single pass 4-throw pupilloplasty for endothelial keratoplasty. *Cornea.* 2017;36:1580-1583.
16. Narang P, Agarwal A, Kumar DA. Single pass four-throw pupilloplasty for angle closure glaucoma. *Indian J Ophthalmol.* 2018; 66(1):120-124.
17. Agarwal A, Narang P, Kumar DA, Agarwal A. Trocar anterior chamber maintainer: improvised infusion technique. *J Cataract Refract Surg.* 2016;42(2):185-189.
18. Kumar DA, Agarwal A, Srinivasan M, Narendrakumar J, Mohanavelu A, Krishnakumar A. Single pass four throw (SFT) pupilloplasty: postoperative mydriasis and fundus visibility in pseudophakic eyes. *J Cataract Refract Surg.* 2017;43(10):1307-1312.

Please visit www.routledge.com/9781630917265

to access additional material.

6

Iridodialysis Repair Management

Richard S. Hoffman, MD; Ashvin Agarwal, MBBS, MS;
Priya Narang, MS; and Amar Agarwal, MS, FRCS, FRCOphth

Keywords

hang-back technique, Hoffman pocket, iridodialysis, iris repair, non-appositional repair, twofold technique, sewing machine technique

The iris root is attached to the sclera and ciliary body, forming the thinnest part of the iris. The disinsertion of the iris root is most commonly traumatic in nature, but it can also be induced iatrogenically.

Indications

- Blunt trauma: Iridodialysis usually occurs due to blunt trauma of an anteroposterior variety—the iris moves back and as it comes forward it disinserts from the root.
- Iatrogenically: The iris is inadvertently pulled by a device or an instrument intracamerally leading to dialysis from the opposite iris.
- Congenital abnormality: In ocular conditions, such as iridocorneal endothelial syndrome, the iris thins and stretches, causing iridodialysis due to the proximity of the stretch to the limbus.

There are various techniques for repair of iridodialysis.[1-11] The following commonly practiced techniques will be discussed in this chapter: hang-back (non-appositional),[12] Hoffman,[13,14] and sewing machine[15,16] and its modified technique (cobbler technique).[17]

Agarwal A, Agarwal A, eds. *Mastering Iris Repair: A Video Textbook of Iris Repair and Pupilloplasty Techniques* (pp 47-58).

Hang-Back (Non-Appositional) Technique

Snyder and Lindsell[12] first described the hang-back technique, which is said to provide a maximal functional and cosmetic outcome to iridodialysis repair.

Principle

This technique works on the principle of hanging the iris on the sclera. A simple analogy is when you place a cloth on a rope and tighten/separate the 2 ends, thereby drawing the cloth back. Here, the iris (cloth) is put on the sutures (ropes) and as you tighten the sutures (ropes) the iris (cloth) moves backward.

This procedure works for 3 clock hours of dialysis or less, beyond that the dialysis warrants a different procedure or 2 hang-back suture passes to be made (see Figures 10-11 through 10-14).

Surgical Procedure

1. Peritomy on the iridodialysis side is fashioned out, and wet cautery is done to cease bleeding.
2. A paracentesis is made diagonally at 4 clock hours from the iridodialysis, and viscoelastic is injected.
3. The pupillary edge of the iris is held using an intracameral forceps. The iris is then stretched to ensure all adhesions are released and the root of the iris is exposed for suture pass.
4. A double-armed 10-0 Prolene (Ethicon) suture is taken. One arm of the suture is passed into the anterior chamber via the paracentesis to the iris root and brought out through the sclera along the plane of the iris. The other side of the suture needle is also passed into the anterior chamber via the same paracentesis (ensuring the needle does not thread the corneal tissue in the path through the paracentesis) and passed into the iris root close to the first iris pass and brought out through the sclera adjacent to the first scleral pass. To be clear, both suture passes are passing through iris root, whole thickness of the sclera, and out.
5. The 2 ends of the suture are now pulled and tied to each other to complete the knot. The knot is then buried into the sclera to prevent any erosion. Utmost care should be taken to ensure that the suture ends are not pulled too much to prevent the overcrowding of the anterior chamber angle structures with the iris tissue.

Advantages

The peripheral iris is left hanging so that creeping of the anterior chamber angle structures with iris tissue is prohibited. This prevents any rise of intraocular pressure.

Because the peripheral iris tissue is not pulled too tightly, corectopia, to a certain extent, is prevented. The disinserted iris sphincter is deprived of its innervation and blood supply. Hence, the tone of the tissue is lessened, which this prevents curling up of the iris tissue.

Hoffman's Technique

Richard Hoffman described this technique that involves making a scleral pocket to bury the suture knots (Figures 6-1 through 6-6).[13,14] It was initially meant for scleral fixation of dislocated intraocular lenses (IOLs). The concept of making the scleral pockets for iridodialysis repair was conceived later (Video 6-1).

Principle

The idea behind this procedure is to prevent erosion of the suture via exposure of the knots and prevent the need of opening the conjunctiva using an intrascleral pocket.

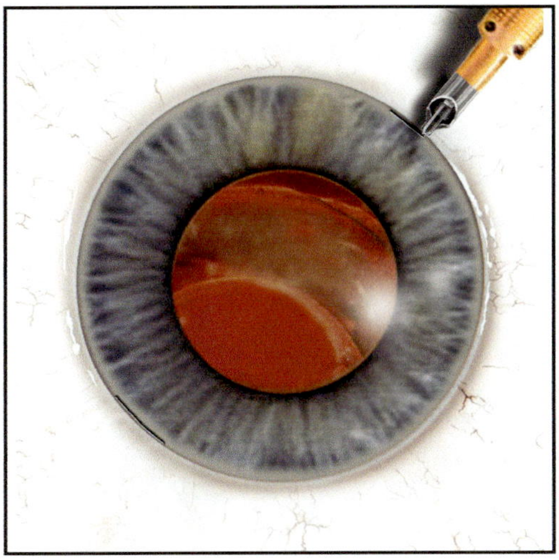

Figure 6-1. Subluxated IOL/capsular bag complex containing Soemmering ring. Two 30-degree long (1 clock hour) and 300- to 400-μm deep clear corneal incisions are made 180 degrees apart with a diamond step knife. These incisions are placed in a meridian that will allow fixation of the lens haptics to the sclera. (Reprinted with permission from Agarwal A, ed. *Mastering Corneal Surgery: Recent Advances and Current Techniques*. Thorofare, NJ: SLACK Incorporated; 2014.)

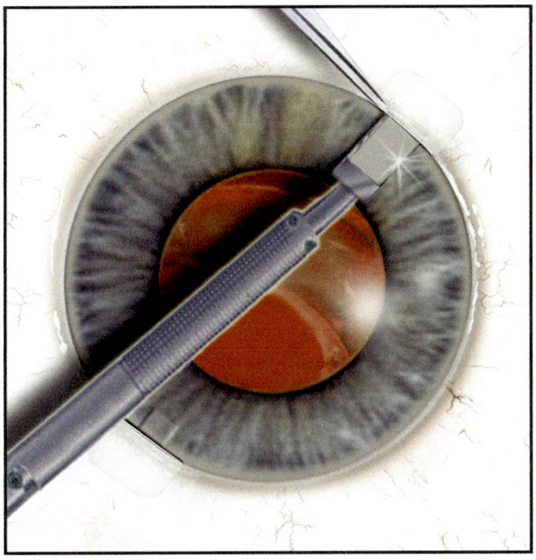

Figure 6-2. Posterior dissection of scleral pockets using a diamond crescent blade. Note the paracentesis originating anterior to the clear corneal incision. (Reprinted with permission from Agarwal A, ed. *Mastering Corneal Surgery: Recent Advances and Current Techniques*. Thorofare, NJ: SLACK Incorporated; 2014.)

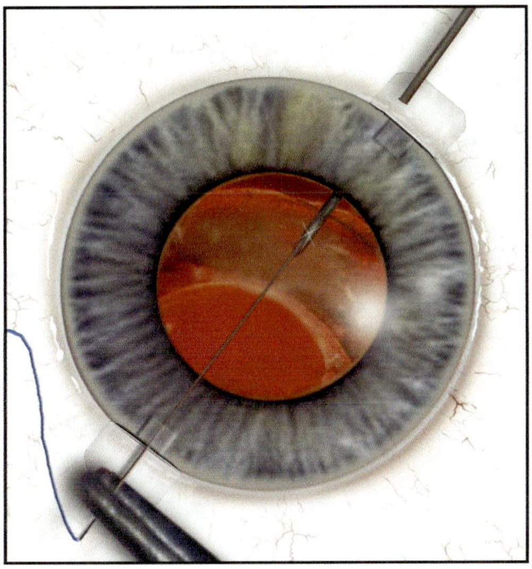

Figure 6-3. Docking of a Prolene suture needle into 27-gauge hollow needle above the capsular bag. The suture needle is passed through the 1-mm paracentesis. The 27-gauge needle is passed into the eye through the conjunctiva and the scleral pocket 1 mm posterior to the surgical limbus. (Reprinted with permission from Agarwal A, ed. *Mastering Corneal Surgery: Recent Advances and Current Techniques*. Thorofare, NJ: SLACK Incorporated; 2014.)

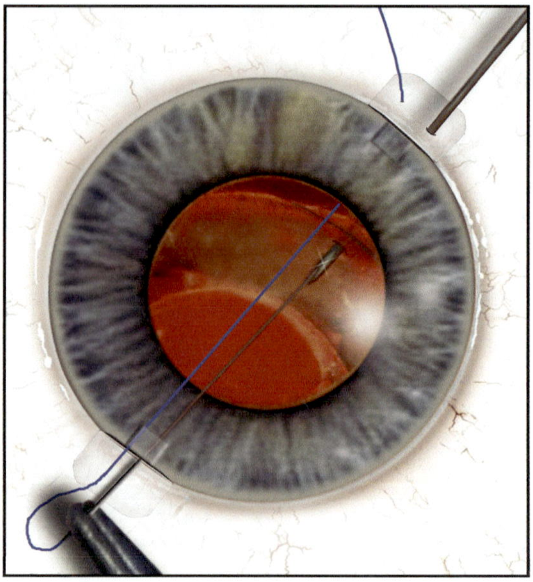

Figure 6-4. Second arm of the double-armed Prolene is inserted through the paracentesis and docked with a second 27-gauge needle that has perforated the capsular bag central to the exposed haptic. (Reprinted with permission from Agarwal A, ed. *Mastering Corneal Surgery: Recent Advances and Current Techniques*. Thorofare, NJ: SLACK Incorporated; 2014.)

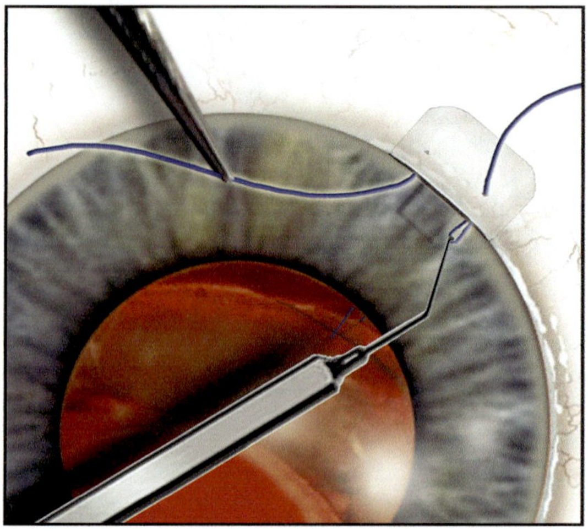

Figure 6-5. Following the second pass of the double-armed suture, the needles are removed and the suture ends are retrieved through the scleral pocket incision using a Sinskey hook. Note the left suture has already been retrieved and is being held with forceps to avoid inadvertent suture loss during retrieval of the right suture. (Reprinted with permission from Agarwal A, ed. *Mastering Corneal Surgery: Recent Advances and Current Techniques*. Thorofare, NJ: SLACK Incorporated; 2014.)

Surgical Procedure

1. It includes making a 350-μm deep clear corneal grooved incision, downward, in the middle third of the iridodialysis for a 3 clock hour iridodialysis or 2 such incisions if the iridodialysis is longer.
2. The incision is then lifted up and a crescent blade helps dissect a pocket toward the fornix in the plane of the sclera without performing a peritomy.
3. A paracentesis is now made 4 clock hours from the iridodialysis site.
4. The pocket margins are marked using a marker on the conjunctiva side to denote its boundaries.
5. One arm of the double-armed 10-0 Prolene suture is now passed through the paracentesis, then passed through the iris root and ab interno brought out through the sclera within the limits of the Hoffman pocket boundary.

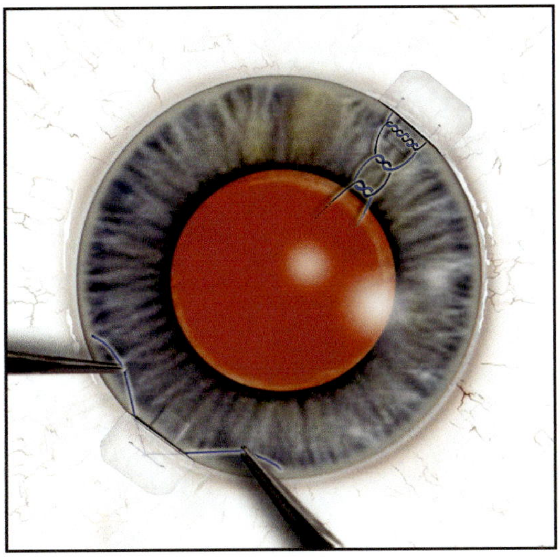

Figure 6-6. Prolene sutures for each haptic are tied allowing the knot to slide under the roof of the scleral pocket. (Reprinted with permission from Agarwal A, ed. *Mastering Corneal Surgery: Recent Advances and Current Techniques*. Thorofare, NJ: SLACK Incorporated; 2014.)

6. The second arm of the suture pass is again passed through the same paracentesis, then passed through the iris root adjacent to the previous pass and brought out of the sclera exactly like the previous pass except that this pass would be adjacent to the previous scleral exit. To be clear, the suture is passing through the iris root, inner sclera, the inside of the Hoffman pocket, outer sclera, subconjunctival space, conjunctiva, and out.
7. Using a Sinskey hook inside the Hoffman pocket via the clear corneal entry of the pocket, both sutures are pulled out.
8. Both suture ends are cut and tied down to a knot. The knot is then slid into the Hoffman pocket and is covered on all sides by sclera inside the pocket.

Advantages

The scleral pocket technique for scleral fixation has several advantages. First, a larger surface area can be created for suture passes than with triangular scleral flaps or scleral grooves. This allows the suture needles to exit anywhere inside the large dissected pocket as long as they are at the appropriate distance from the surgical limbus (0.5 to 1 mm for ciliary sulcus fixation). This is especially useful when using an ab interno approach. Second, dissection of the scleral pocket initiated from a clear corneal incision avoids the need for conjunctival dissection or scleral cautery. This should cause less discomfort in patients undergoing procedures with topical anesthesia where unforeseen complications may necessitate the use of scleral fixated lenses or fixated capsular bag prostheses. The dissection of the distal scleral pocket is also easier to perform than a triangular flap in the distal location because the dissection can proceed directed away from the surgeon in a slightly "downhill" direction. In addition, the procedure may be expedited, relative to a triangular flap technique, because conjunctival dissection is avoided and a sutured wound close is unnecessary. Finally, less astigmatism may be induced than would occur with the placement of 2 radial sutures through each of 2 opposing triangular flaps in the same meridian. Although 2 opposed 30-degree vertical clear corneal incisions do have a small flattening effect in the meridian of placement, the small arc length and relatively superficial depth compared to traditional limbal relaxing incisions induces very little astigmatic effect. This can be modified by using more superficial 300-µm incisions depending on the desired astigmatic result.

Using a scleral pocket with hook-retrieval of the suture ends can be performed for any procedure requiring transscleral fixation. This includes implantation of secondary IOLs, repair of dislocated IOLs, employment of adjunctive surgical devices, such as Ahmed Capsular Tension Segments (FCI Ophthalmics) and Cionni Capsular Tension Rings (FCI Ophthalmics), and repair of iridodialyses. This modification of the traditional scleral flap allows for a simpler creation of

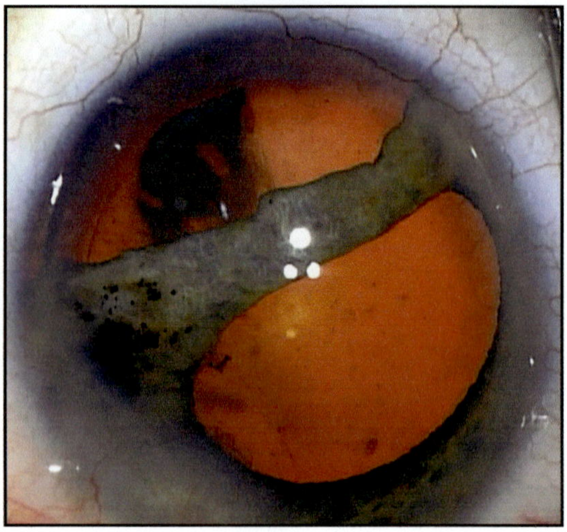

Figure 6-7. Intraoperative view of a 120-degree nasal iridodialysis. (Reprinted with permission from Agarwal A, ed. *Mastering Corneal Surgery: Recent Advances and Current Techniques*. Thorofare, NJ: SLACK Incorporated; 2014.)

a scleral covering negating the need to rotate suture knots while facilitating needle placement for either an ab interno or ab externo technique.

In short, the basic advantages can be summarized as follows:

- Scleral cauterization and collagen denaturation are avoided.
- Extrusion of the suture knot is avoided as it gets buried in the scleral wall.
- Because conjunctival dissection is not performed, patients with filtering blebs or patients with glaucoma, who may require surgery in future, are at an additional advantage.

Iridodialysis Repair Through a Scleral Pocket

Repair of the traumatic iridodialysis can be accomplished by means of single or multiple McCannel sutures through an ab externo approach or using one or more double-armed sutures with an ab interno approach. When fixating anything to the sclera, it is important to rotate the suture knots into the sclera or cover the suture knots under a scleral flap to prevent erosion of the overlying conjunctiva that could then allow for the development of endophthalmitis. Although suture knot rotation is relatively simple and straightforward, an alternative method of repairing a traumatic iridodialysis uses one or more sclera pockets that eliminate the need for a conjunctival peritomy while still enabling covering of the suture knot without the need for knot rotation.

If the iridodialysis is 3 clock hours or less, 1 double-armed Prolene suture and 1 pocket is all that is required. For larger dialyses, 2 pockets will be needed (Figure 6-7). The first step is to place a 350-µm deep grooved incision at the clear cornea limbus overlying the middle third of the dialysis. For large dialyses, 2 grooves of 2 clock hour lengths are placed. Each grooved incision is then dissected posteriorly in the plane of the sclera for approximately 2 mm to create a scleral pocket. Using a metal crescent blade and lifting up on the posterior edge of the grooved incision during the dissection facilitates creation of the scleral pocket. Once the pockets are dissected, the conjunctival surface overlying the lateral extent of each pocket is marked with gentian violet to assist in suture needle placement.

A paracentesis is then made 3 to 4 clock hours from the site of fixation and viscoelastic is injected into the anterior chamber. A 10-0 Prolene suture on a double-armed CIF-4 needle (Ethicon) is passed through the paracentesis, incorporating the edge of the dialysed iris root at one-third the lateral distance from the attached edge of the iris root. The needle is then passed through the full-thickness of the globe, exiting approximately 2 mm posterior to the limbus within the area of the dissected pocket. The second arm of the double-armed suture is passed through the same paracentesis, through the iris root edge, 3 mm adjacent to the first pass, and out through the sclera 2 to 3 mm adjacent to the first pass and 2 mm posterior to the limbus. It is better to err on passing the needle posterior to the original insertion rather than anterior to avoid obstructing the trabecular meshwork.

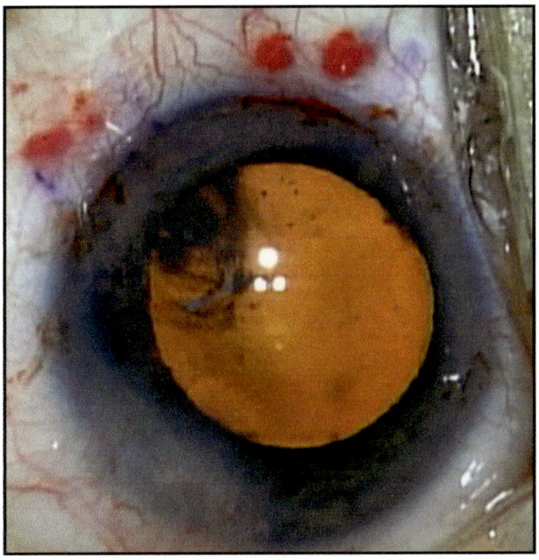

Figure 6-8. Appearance of a dilated pupil following iridodialysis repair and prior to phacoemulsification. (Reprinted with permission from Agarwal A, ed. *Mastering Corneal Surgery: Recent Advances and Current Techniques*. Thorofare, NJ: SLACK Incorporated; 2014.)

Wiggling the needle tip back and forth as it goes through the paracentesis will avoid accidently passing the suture needle through corneal stroma. Placing the viscoelastic cannula into the paracentesis to hold the paracentesis open while passing the needle into the anterior chamber will also facilitate entry if this step becomes difficult. For a single pocket dialysis of less than 90 degrees, the 2 needle passes should basically trisect the dialysis into thirds. After the sutures have been placed, the needles are removed, and the suture ends are retrieved through the external opening of the scleral pocket by placing a Sinskey hook into the pocket and pulling each suture end out. After both suture ends of the double-armed suture have been externalized, the suture is tightened and tied, allowing the knot to slide under the protective roof of the scleral pocket. The suture ends are then trimmed and no additional wound closure of the pockets is required (Figure 6-8).

These repairs are usually performed in combination with cataract extraction. It is best to repair the iridodialysis before phacoemulsification to facilitate access to the lens and avoid inadvertent aspiration and enlargement of the iridodialysis. Following phacoemulsification, IOL implantation, and viscoelastic removal, the pupil should be constricted intraoperatively to determine if significant corectopia has been created from the iridodialysis repair. If so, a single suture can be placed through the pupillary margin, using a Siepser slip-knot technique, to pinch the pupil into a rounder and smaller size if desired.

Sewing Machine Technique

Principle

This technique[15-17] derives its name from a sewing machine that is used to stitch clothes. The tip of the needle has a running thread through it at all times. With cloth under the needle, the stitching process begins by piercing the cloth and moving to an adjacent site, thereby binding both pieces together with a stitch. This same concept is taken and applied to iris (cloth) and sclera (the base it binds to).

Surgical Procedure

The Setup

Before beginning the procedure, the surgeon must prepare the instrument because the instrument does not come pre-prepared from the manufacturer. This involves threading of a 10-0 Prolene suture into a 26-gauge needle two-thirds of the way (Video 6-2). This now behaves as your sewing machine needle.

The Surgery

1. A peritomy is performed on the side of the iridodialysis, and a wet cautery is performed to achieve hemostasis.
2. A scleral tunnel is made along the iridodialysis at the iris plane.
3. A paracentesis is made opposite to the iridodialysis.
4. The previously prepared instrument (the 26-gauge needle threaded with the 10-0 Prolene suture) is now passed through the paracentesis ab interno, passing the tip of the 26-gauge needle through the iris root on the opposite side and out through the scleral tunnel.
5. The free end of the Prolene suture is pulled out from the scleral tunnel and left to lie outside, while the 26-gauge needle is retracted inside the eye and passed through an adjacent site on the iris root and brought out through the scleral tunnel adjacent to the first pass. At this time, a loop is pulled out through the tip of the 26-gauge needle.
6. This process is continued until the iridodialysis is covered.
7. The 26-gauge needle is then retracted outside the eye and the Prolene suture tip is cut where the loops are protruding out from the scleral tunnel except for one free end of the Prolene suture (that of the first pass).
8. The loops are then cut right in the middle, and the suture ends are now numbered (1, 2, 3, 4, 5, etc)
9. The alternate sutures (1 and 2, 2 and 3, 3 and 4) are then tightened and tied down, and the knot is buried into the scleral tunnel to prevent erosion.
10. This completes the sewing machine technique of iridodialysis repair (Figures 6-9 and 6-10).

Other Techniques

Iridodialysis repair includes procedures that have been tried in the past, such as the following:

- Sutureless technique for iridodialysis repair: The procedure involved performing a peritomy on the side of the iridodialysis, making 3 to 4 sclerotomies close to each other at the iris plane, and pulling the iris root out using microvitreoretinal forceps, thereby plugging the sclerotomy. The area is then covered with conjunctiva. Though the procedure is simple, it can have complications, such as endophthalmitis.
- External approach to iridodialysis repair: A peritomy is fashioned out at the site of the iridodialysis. Then a limbal clear corneal wound is fashioned, and the iris root is pulled out of the clear corneal incision. A 10-0 Prolene double-armed suture is passed through the iris root adjacent to each other and a loop is created on top of the iris. The iris is then placed in the anterior chamber and a suture is passed inside out from the anterior chamber to the external sclera and a knot is tied outside. The knot is then buried into the sclera to prevent erosion or, alternatively, this can be done under a flap or a Hoffman pocket.

Complications of Iridodialysis Repair

Complications can include the following:

- Bleeding
- Extension of iris root tear
- Peeking pupil
- Erosion of suture material: This usually happens when we leave a suture knot exposed under the conjunctiva. Hence, it's a good idea to bury the suture or use a scleral flap or a Hoffman's pocket to cover the suture knot.
- Lens touch in case of phakic eye: To avoid this complication, lens extraction is usually performed simultaneously.

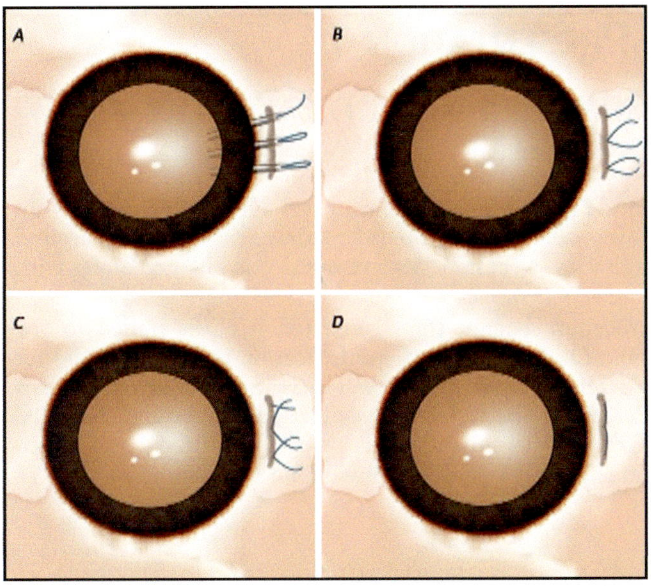

Figure 6-9. Illustration of sewing machine technique. (A) Suture loops are pulled from the scleral side along the entire length of iridodialysis. (B) The suture loops are cut. (C) Adjacent suture threads are tied to each other. (D) Iridodialysis repair is complete.

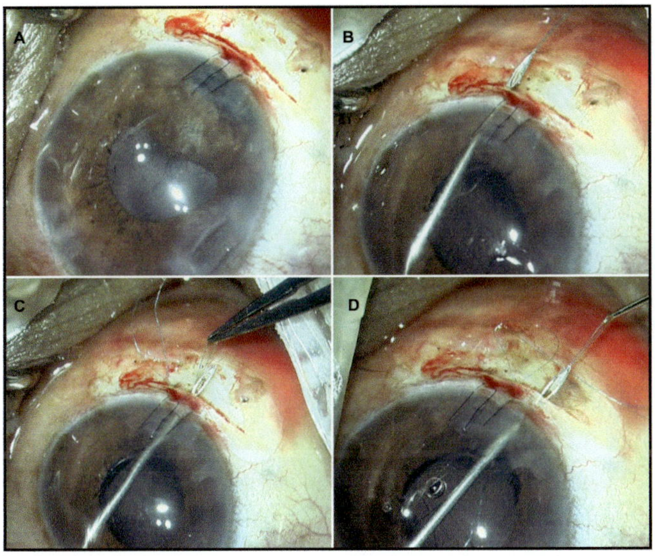

Figure 6-10. Clinical image of sewing machine technique. (A) Moderate amount of iridodialysis. A scleral groove is made along the entire extent of iris disinsertion. (B) The threaded 26-gauge needle is passed from the opposite paracentesis into the anterior chamber engaging the peripheral part of disinserted iris. (C, D) The suture loop is withdrawn and similar attempts are repeated until the iridodialysis portion is covered. The suture loops are then cut and adjacent suture loops tied. The iridodialysis repair is complete.

Discussion

Of the various techniques available for iridodialysis repair, the surgeon should chose the technique that he or she is comfortable with. Often, a combination of techniques is necessary for iridodialysis repair.[18] Before the surgeon begins performing the surgical procedure, the essential surgical tools should be prepared.

The iris tissue is a very flexible. Surgeons should handle the tissue very delicately and consider the amount of iris that needs to be involved for repair. Using a large area of iris tissue in the needle may lead to the iris being drawn to one side, or corectopia. Alternatively, involving too little of the iris tissue in the needle could lead to the suture cutting through the iris, which means the procedure would need to be repeated.

Iridodialysis repair has excellent cosmetic and functional outcomes. Surgeons should master the repair techniques for the benefit of their patients.

Case Presentation 1

Sewing Machine Technique for Iridodialysis Repair

Ashvin Agarwal, MBBS, MS

A male patient aged 56 years presented with dimness of vision and a history of trauma. On slit-lamp examination, an iridodialysis was seen in the temporal quadrant that extended around 70 to 80 degrees. Because the patient also has a cataract, lens removal was planned along with the iridodialysis repair.

Before the phacoemulsification procedure began, the disinserted iris was pulled to the temporal side by implanting an iris hook. During the phacoemulsification procedure, posterior capsular dehiscence was observed. Therefore, a vitrectomy was performed followed by lens removal and glued intrascleral fixation. After the secured lens fixation, the sewing machine technique was performed, which affixed the iris tissue to its base (Figure 6-11 and Video 6-3). Postoperatively, the patient regained good visual acuity with no complaints of glare or photophobia.

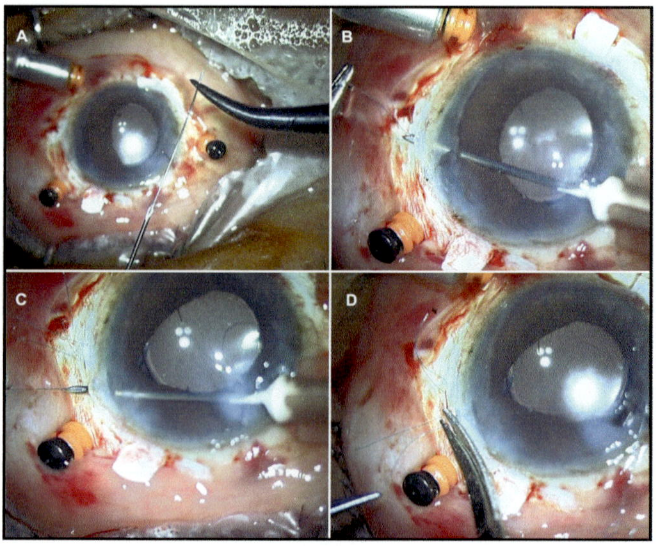

Figure 6-11. Sewing machine technique for iridodialysis repair. (A) The 10-0 suture needle is threaded in to the barrel of a 26-gauge needle. (B) The 26-gauge needle threaded with the 10-0 Prolene suture is now passed through the paracentesis ab interno, passing the tip of the 26-gauge needle through the iris root on the opposite side and out through the scleral tunnel. (C) The free end of the Prolene suture is pulled out from the scleral tunnel and left to lie outside, while the 26-gauge needle is retracted inside the eye and passed through an adjacent site on the iris root and brought out through the scleral tunnel adjacent to the first pass. At this time, a loop is pulled out through the tip of the 26-gauge needle. (D) The loop is then cut right in the middle. The alternate sutures are then tightened and tied down.

Case Presentation 2

Modified Sewing Machine Technique for Iridodialysis Repair, Intraocular Lens Relocation, Iris Coloboma Repair, Cionni Ring Fixation, and Scleral Fixated Intraocular Lens

Ravi Kumar K V, PGDO, FCO (LVPEI), FICO (SWISS)

Sewing machine technique for iridodialysis repair is based on the principle of how a sewing machine functions and uses a pre-threaded 26-gauge needle with 10-0 Prolene suture in a closed chamber. This technique is made simpler by using only one knot for the entire iris dialysis repair. Modified sewing machine technique can also tackle other clinical conditions/procedures like IOL subluxation, iris coloboma, zonular dialysis using Cionni Capsular Tension Rings, and a scleral fixated IOL. It is a cost-effective, innovative, minimally invasive, easy-to-learn procedure with the potential to tackle several problems related with cataract surgery, trauma, and iris defects. A cataract surgeon can learn to perform this procedure (Figure 6-12 and Video 6-4).[15,17]

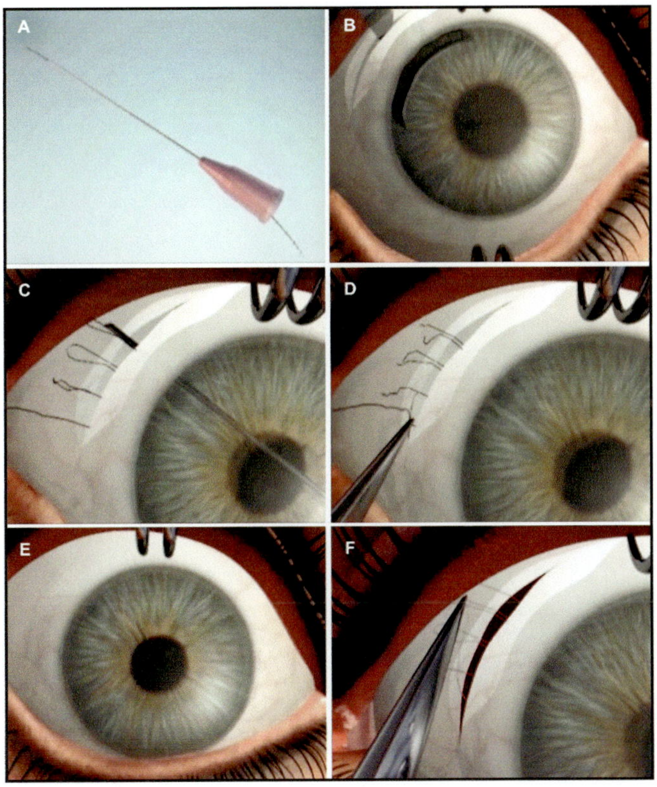

Figure 6-12. Modified sewing machine technique for iridodialysis. (A) Cut the needle of 10-0 Prolene suture and remove the needle. Retrograde threading of 10-0 Prolene suture into 26-gauge needle. (B) Create a partial-thickness scleral tunnel parallel to and all along the iris dialysis (2 mm away from the limbus). Then perform pupil constriction by pilocarpine. (C) Create suture loops like sewing machine stitches all along the dialysis by passing a pre-threaded 26-gauge needle with the suture through the root of iris dialysis and scleral tunnel from inside out several times. (D) Cut the loops of Prolene and tie the adjacent free ends to each other so that the knots get buried into scleral tunnel. (E) Close the conjunctiva using 10-0 nylon or vicryl or bipolar cautery. (F) In the modified sewing machine technique, after creating suture loops as described earlier, the first free end of the suture is passed through the loops and tied with the second free end of suture so that only one knot is sufficient for the entire iris dialysis repair.

References

1. Richards JC, Kennedy CJ. Sutureless technique for repair of traumatic iridodialysis. *Ophthalmic Surg Lasers Imaging.* 2006;37:508-510.
2. Erakgun T, Kaskaloglu M, Kayikcioglu O. A simple closed chamber technique for repair of traumatic iridodialysis in phakic eyes. *Ophthalmic Surg Lasers.* 2001;32:83-85.
3. Brown SM. A technique for repair of iridodialysis in children. *JAAPOS.* 1998;2:380-382.
4. Wachler BB, Krueger RR. Double-armed McCannel suture for repair of traumatic iridodialysis. *Am J Ophthalmol.* 1996;122:109-110.
5. Viestenz A, Kuchle M. Ocular contusion caused by elastic cords: a retrospective analysis using the Erlangen Ocular Contusion Registry. *Clin Experiment Ophthalmol.* 2002;30:266-269
6. McCannel MA. A retrievable suture idea for anterior uveal problems. *Ophthalmic Surg.* 1976;7:98-103
7. Kaufman SC, Insler MS. Surgical repair of a traumatic iridodialysis. *Ophthalmic Surg Lasers.* 1996;27:963-966
8. Bardak Y, Ozerturk Y, Durmus M, Mensiz E, Aytuluner E. Closed chamber iridodialysis repair using a needle with a distal hole. *J Cataract Refract Surg.* 2000;26:173-176
9. Zeiter JH, Shin DH, Shi DX. A closed chamber technique for repair of iridodialysis. *Ophthalmic Surg.* 1993;24:476-480
10. Nunziata BR. Repair of iridodialysis using a 17-millimeter straight needle. *Ophthalmic Surg Lasers.* 1993;24:627-629
11. Silva JL, Povoa J, Lobo C, Murta J. New technique for iridodialysis correction: single-knot sewing-machine suture. *J Cataract Refract Surg.* 2016;42:520-523.
12. Snyder ME, Lindsell LB. Nonappositional repair of iridodialysis. *J Cataract Refract Surg.* 2011;37:625-628.
13. Hoffman RS, Fine IH, Packer M. Scleral fixation without conjunctival dissection. *J Cataract Refract Surg.* 2006;32:1907-1912.
14. Hoffman RS. Iridodialysis repair through a scleral pocket. *Eye World News.* www.eyeworld.org/article-iridodialysis-repair-through-a-scleral-pocket. Published July 2011. Accessed April 27, 2020.
15. Kumar KVR. Sewing machine technique for iridodialysis repair. *Delhi Journal of Ophthalmology.* 2014;24:248-251.
16. Safran SG. Sewing machine style technique for iridodialysis repair. *Ocular Surgery News.* 1995;49.
17. Kumar KVR. Modified sewing machine technique for iridodialysis repair, intraocular lens relocation, iris coloboma repair, Cionni ring fixation, and scleral-fixated intraocular lens. *Indian J Ophthalmol.* 2018;66(8):1169-1176.
18. Narang P, Agarwal A, Agarwal A, Agarwal A. Twofold technique of nonappositional repair with single-pass four-throw pupilloplasty for iridodialysis. *J Cataract Refract Surg.* 2018;44(12):1413-1420.

Please visit www.routledge.com/9781630917265 to access additional material.

SECTION II

IRIS REPAIR AND PUPILLOPLASTY SPECIAL TOPICS

7

Pupilloplasty in Special Indications

Urrets-Zavalia Syndrome and Secondary Glaucoma

Priya Narang, MS, and Amar Agarwal, MS, FRCS, FRCOphth

KEYWORDS

angle-closure glaucoma, deep anterior lamellar keratoplasty, penetrating keratoplasty, peripheral anterior synechia, pupilloplasty, secondary glaucoma, single-pass four-throw pupilloplasty, Urrets-Zavalia syndrome

URRETS-ZAVALIA SYNDROME

In 1963, Urrets-Zavalia described a clinical condition following a penetrating keratoplasty surgery that was later named Urrets-Zavalia syndrome.[1] A persistently dilated pupil in the postoperative period characterizes the syndrome that may be associated with raised intraocular pressure (IOP) along with patches of iris atrophy. Although the actual etiopathogenesis is unknown, it is believed that a persistently dilated pupil causes mechanical blockage of the anterior chamber angle and eventually leads to formation of peripheral anterior synechia (PAS) followed by secondary angle closure (Figure 7-1). Following its initial description in a case with penetrating keratoplasty, it has been subsequently described postoperatively in cases with trabeculectomy,[2] argon laser peripheral iridoplasty,[3] phakic anterior chamber intraocular lens (IOL) implantation,[4-6] deep anterior lamellar keratoplasty,[7-10] Descemet's stripping automated endothelial keratoplasty,[11-13] goniotomy,[14] octafluoropropane injection (C_3F_8),[15] and glued intrascleral fixation of IOL.[16] The persistently dilated pupil in Urrets-Zavalia syndrome fails to respond to miotics, sympatholytic agents, or to alpha-adrenergic blockers. Therefore, the treatment is directed mainly toward control of glare and photophobia. Surgical pupilloplasty can be considered for these cases as it helps to provide symptomatic relief to the patients (Video 7-1).[16]

Agarwal A, Agarwal A, eds. *Mastering Iris Repair: A Video Textbook of Iris Repair and Pupilloplasty Techniques* (pp 61-70).

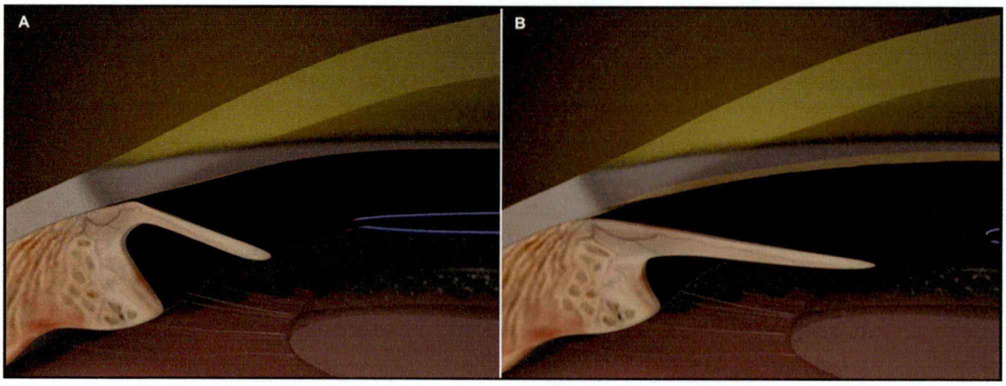

Figure 7-1. Illustration describing the mechanism of action of surgical pupilloplasty. (A) The image depicts narrow angle structures. A 10-0 suture for performing pupilloplasty is passed through the iris tissue along the pupillary border. (B) Postoperatively, the angle structures open up because the mechanical blockage is relieved by the peripheral pull of the iris tissue.

Surgical Consideration

Certain aspects should be taken into consideration while performing pupilloplasty in a case with Urrets-Zavalia syndrome as there is associated iris atrophy, and the iris is often inflexible. Therefore, pupillary stretching is recommended as an initial step. This is performed by holding the pupil margin with blunt end-opening forceps and slowly pulling the iris tissue toward the pupil centre. This maneuver helps to assess the flexibility of the iris tissue, and it also provides an estimate of the amount of iris tissue that can be incorporated into the needle to perform a pupilloplasty procedure. All measures should be taken to prevent passing the needle through or from the area adjacent to the iris atrophy patch because doing so would lead to gaping and cutting through the iris tissue.

Angle-Closure Glaucoma and Secondary Glaucoma

Angle-closure glaucoma (ACG) is characterized by narrow anterior chamber angles with raised IOP and associated field defects with or without a pupillary block. PAS are often present and lead to further narrowing of angle structures. Laser peripheral iridectomy relieves the pupillary block mechanism, and argon laser peripheral iridoplasty relieves the mechanical blockage by pulling the peripheral iris tissue. In selected cases of secondary glaucoma associated with silicon oil tamponade, mechanical changes are induced in the trabecular meshwork that lead to fibrosis of the meshwork eventually leading to raised IOP and formation of PAS.[17] As soon as the patient reports raised IOP, removal of the silicon oil is indicated in these cases as delaying it to a later stage is risky. Patients with silicon oil have an associated posterior segment pathology; therefore, the surgeon should consider this before a silicon oil removal is planned (Figure 7-2).

Surgical Consideration

Pupillary stretching is recommended in cases with ACG, as it facilitates breaking of the PAS due to the mechanical pull of the iris tissue. The pupilloplasty procedure should be performed under fluid infusion. An ophthalmic viscosurgical device (OVDs) should be avoided because these cases are associated with raised IOP. Also, fluid is the natural milieu of the eye so it is preferred to an OVD. In addition to this, a greater amount of iris tissue should be involved in the 10-0 suture needle, as substantial amount of stretch is necessary to induce the breakage of PAS. A multiple quadrant approach should be adopted, and the number of quadrants involved depends on the degree of PAS detected on gonioscopy. For PAS greater than 270 degrees, a 6-point traction (3 quadrant approach) is necessary; whereas for less than 270 degrees of PAS, a 4-point traction (2 quadrant approach) is sufficient (Figure 7-3).

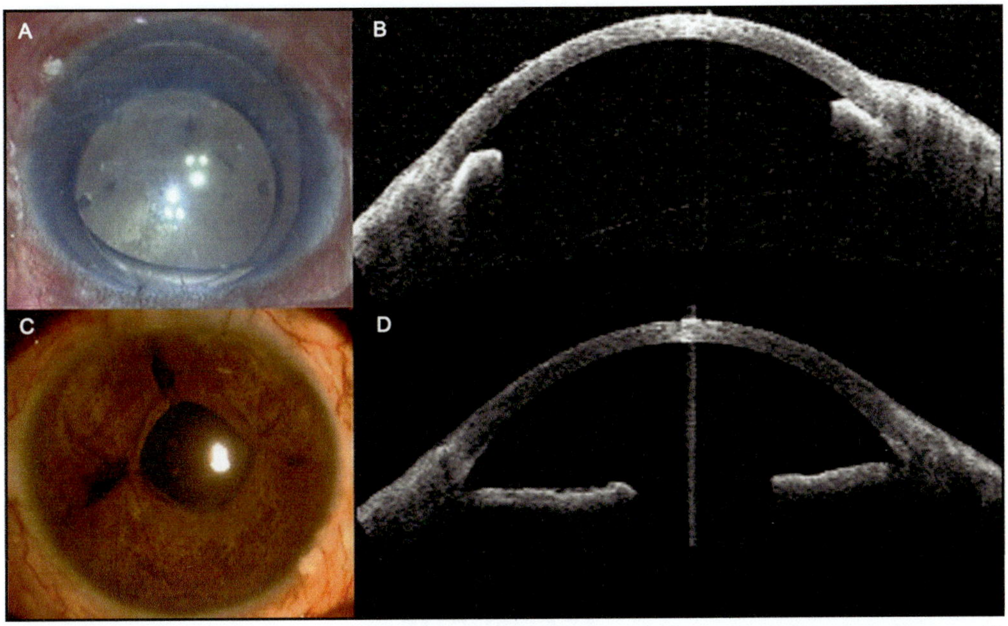

Figure 7-2. Clinical image of a case with secondary glaucoma due to silicon oil. (A) Pseudophakic eye with presence of silicon oil in anterior chamber and decompensated cornea. (B) AS-OCT denoting narrow angle structures. (C) Postoperative image following SFT pupilloplasty. A 3 quadrant approach was chosen and a 6-point traction was performed. (D) AS-OCT denoting open angles in postoperative period.

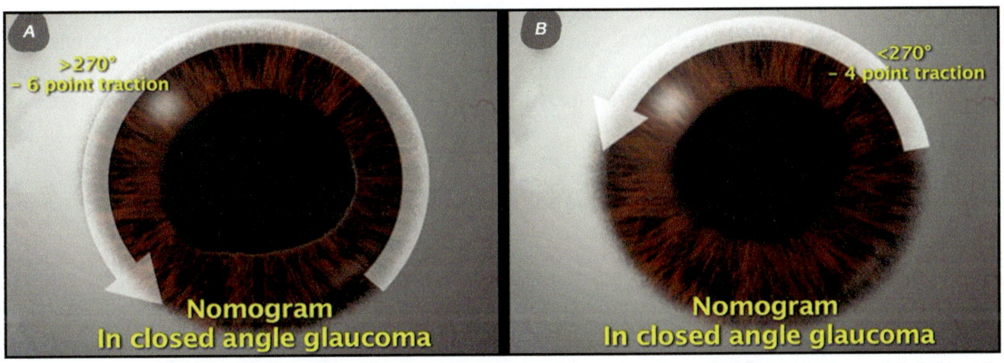

Figure 7-3. Illustration depicting the nomogram for performing surgical pupilloplasty in cases with ACG with PAS. (A) In eyes with more than 270 degrees of PAS, a 6-point traction is advised (ie, the patient undergoes pupilloplasty in 3 quadrants). (B) In eyes with less than 270 degrees PAS, a 4-point traction is advised (ie the patient undergoes pupilloplasty in 2 quadrants).

Investigations

In addition to obtaining ocular history and recording best-corrected Snellen's visual acuity in the preoperative and postoperative follow-ups, a detailed slit-lamp examination of the anterior segment and Goldmann applanation tonometry to measure the IOP should be performed in all the cases.

In these cases, the role of gonioscopy should not be underestimated. The anterior chamber angles should be assessed using a 3-mirror Goldmann-type gonioscopy lens (Volk Optical) in primary gaze. Indentation gonioscopy should be performed to determine whether the angle closure is due to apposition or due to PAS. The authors prefer to use a Zeiss-style 4-mirror gonioscopy. Performing an intraoperative gonioscopy, which gives a direct view of the opening of the angles during the surgical procedure, is optional in these cases. Anterior segment optical coherence

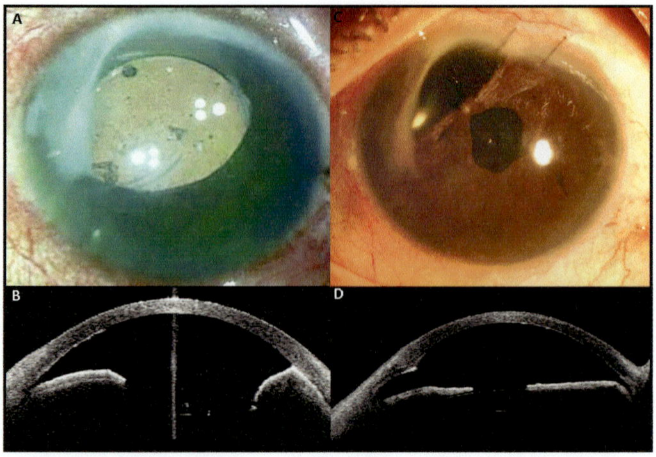

Figure 7-4. SFT pupilloplasty in ACG. (A) ACG. (B) AS-OCT shows a closed angle. (C) Angle open following SFT pupilloplasty. (D) AS-OCT shows angle open after SFT pupilloplasty.

tomography (AS-OCT) serves as an additional tool to document the opening of the angles in the preoperative and postoperative period.

Technique

Taking all the surgical aspects into consideration, the authors adopted the single-pass four-throw (SFT) pupilloplasty technique for cases with Urrets-Zavalia syndrome and secondary angle closure due to various advantages associated with the procedure.[16-18] First, the SFT technique involves a single pass made from the anterior chamber compared to the Siepser and McCannel methods. Therefore, there is minimal anterior chamber manipulation that likely translates into less inflammation in the postoperative period. Second, the SFT technique is simple, fast, and easy to emulate. All surgeons who are accustomed to performing a Siepser or a McCannel method can easily adopt it (Figure 7-4).

Discussion

ACG is one of the major causes of blindness worldwide for which specific medical and surgical modalities of treatment have been defined. Laser peripheral iridectomy and argon laser peripheral iridoplasty are often indicated. Despite this, the raised IOP fails to respond to the laser procedures and the ACG progresses unabated. Goniosynechialysis in association with iris encerclage has been proposed as a line of treatment in refractory angle closure for atonic pupil and prevention of glare and photophobia. The role of surgical pupilloplasty in select cases of ACG has been recently documented by the authors with favorable outcomes.[19] However, the authors would recommend performing a surgical pupilloplasty along with removal of the natural lens and placement of a foldable IOL. This creates additional space in the anterior chamber and facilitates the opening of the angle to a certain extent. Selective to cases with plateau iris syndrome, laser peripheral iridectomy works seldom and argon laser peripheral iridoplasty is often indicated. SFT pupilloplasty has been reported to work efficiently in these cases (Figures 7-5 through 7-8).

In cases with Urrets-Zavalia syndrome, cosmetic contact lenses do not offer a permanent solution to the clinical condition. Surgical pupilloplasty not only helps to relive the symptoms of glare/photophobia but also helps by breaking the PAS and controlling the rise of IOP. Nevertheless, it should be stated that surgical pupilloplasty should be performed in the initial stages when the PAS have begun to form and before the trabecular meshwork is distorted due to fibrosis. Performing the procedure at a later stage would not be beneficial, as aqueous drainage would not be facilitated if fibrosis of the trabecular meshwork were advanced beyond a certain extent.

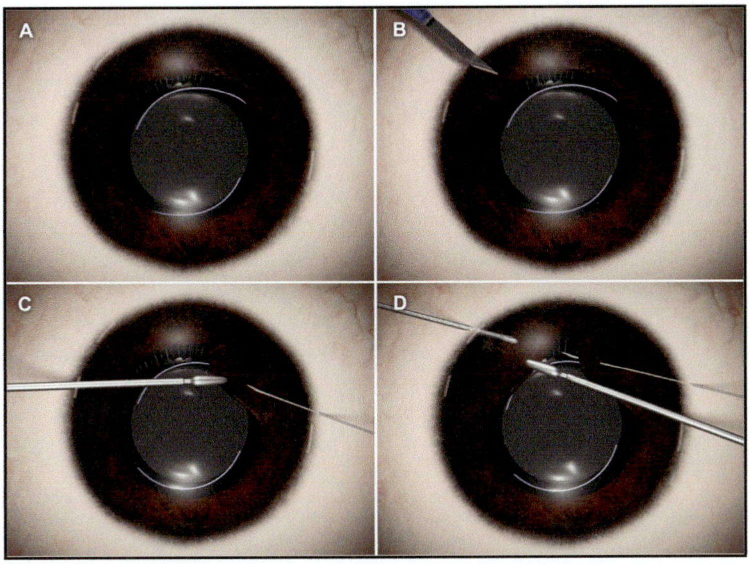

Figure 7-5. Part 1: A step-by-step SFT pupilloplasty. (A) A pseudophakic eye needing pupilloplasty. During the procedure, use a trocar anterior chamber maintainer or anterior chamber maintainer for continuous fluid infusion in the eye. An OVD may also be used, but if hyphema occurs during the procedure, it cannot be washed away. (B) Paracentesis made to create a clear corneal incision. (C) Prolene suture with needle enters the clear cornea and then pierces the iris. Note that the glued IOL forceps holds the iris while the needle is piercing the iris so that no trauma, such as an iridodialysis, occurs. (D) A 26- or 30-gauge needle enters the clear corneal incision site and pierces the iris. Once again, the glued IOL forceps holds the iris while this maneuver is being performed to make the procedure easy and safe.

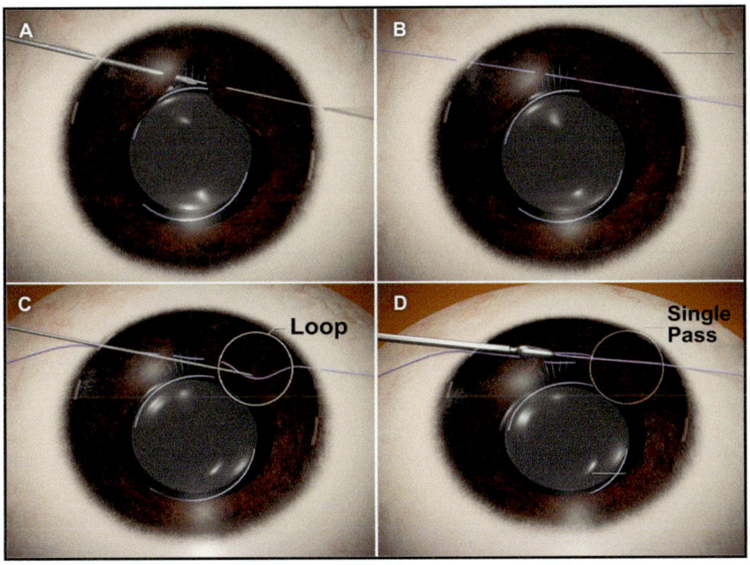

Figure 7-6. Part 2: A step-by-step SFT pupilloplasty. (A) Railroad technique is performed. The Prolene suture is passed through the 26- or 30-gauge needle. (B) The suture is then passed out through the clear corneal incision. (C) A loop is created. This is the single pass. (D) The loop is grasped with the glued IOL forceps to bring it out through the clear corneal incision.

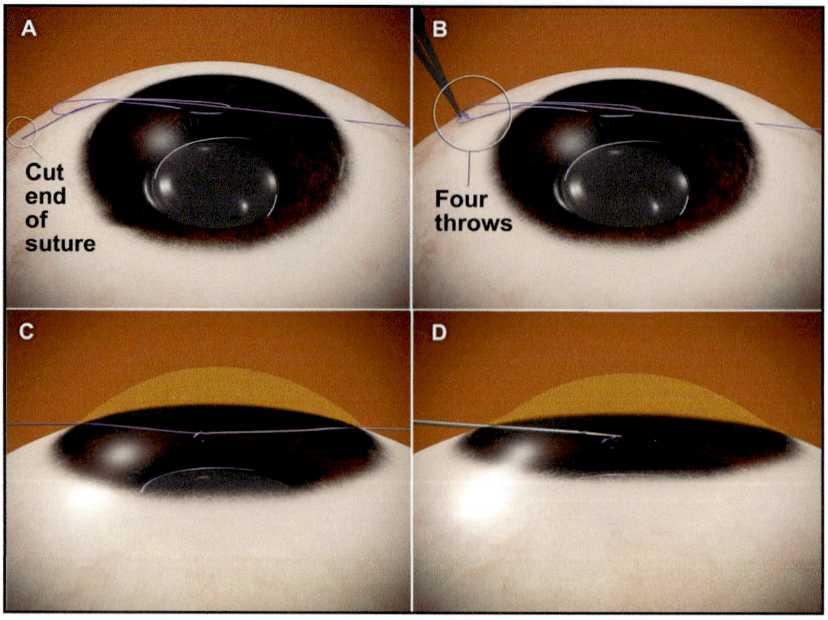

Figure 7-7. Part 3: A step-by-step SFT pupilloplasty. (A) The loop is brought out through the clear corneal incision. (B) The cut end of the suture is passed 4 times through the loop. This is the 4 throws. (C) The 2 ends of the suture are now pulled and the helical lock on the iris created by the suture. (D) The suture ends are cut by microscissors.

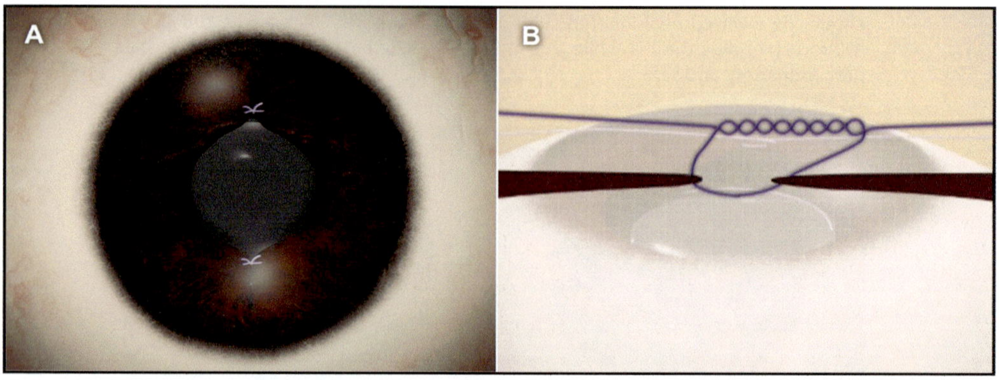

Figure 7-8. Part 4: A step-by-step SFT pupilloplasty. (A) The same procedure can be performed on the other side of the pupil to make a small pupil. It can be performed many times in different areas depending on what is being treated—mydriasis, ACG, or creating a pinhole pupilloplasty for high irregular astigmatism. (B) The helical knot created by the SFT pupilloplasty technique.

Case Presentation 1

Urrets-Zavalia Syndrome Post Penetrating Keratoplasty

Priya Narang, MS and Amar Agarwal, MS, FRCS, FRCOphth

A male patient aged 45 years presented with a history of surgical procedure of penetrating keratoplasty along with cataract extraction. The initial postoperative period was uneventful. After 4 weeks, the patient developed pain in the eye along with decreased visual acuity. On clinical examination, the IOP was raised (45 mm Hg) and the pupil was fully dilated (no history of instilling a mydriatic). It was difficult to assess the angle structures on gonioscopy due to associated corneal haze and the rim of the penetrating keratoplasty graft occluding the view on the gonioscopy mirror. AS-OCT revealed narrowing of the angle structures.

The IOP was controlled with acetazolamide (carbonic anhydrase inhibitor) tablets 3 times per day along with alpha agonists. A drop of pilocarpine 1% (parasympathomimetic) was instilled in the eye to check for pupillary constriction. A clinical diagnosis of Urrets-Zavalia syndrome was made when the pupil failed to respond to the topical drop.

An SFT pupilloplasty was performed in 3 quadrants inducing a 6-point traction. Postoperatively, the corneal haze cleared. IOP was 18 mm Hg on postoperative day 7 and 10 mm Hg at the 1-month postoperative follow-up. AS-OCT revealed opening of the angle structures. The patient's visual acuity improved to 20/60 with the IOP maintained at 10 mm Hg at the 6 month follow-up. There was no incidence of glare or photophobia, or any other untoward event in the postoperative period (Figure 7-9).

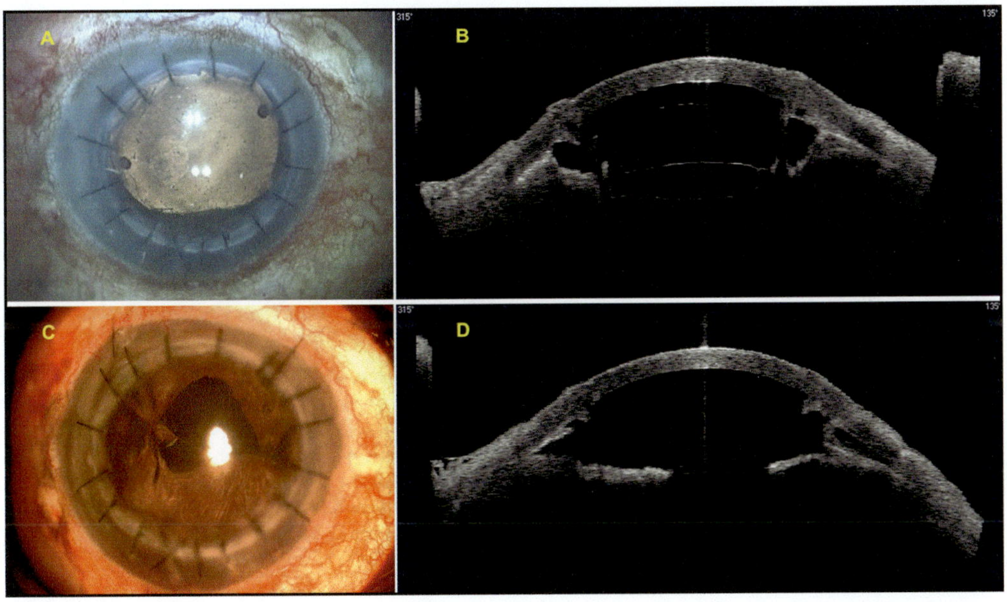

Figure 7-9. Cases of Urrets-Zavalia syndrome. (A, C) Case 1 and case 2 of Urrets-Zavalia syndrome following a penetrating keratoplasty procedure. (B, D) Postoperative image of both the cases with AS-OCT demonstrating opening of angles.

Case Presentation 2

Surgical Pupilloplasty in Angle-Closure Glaucoma

Amar Agarwal, MS, FRCS, FRCOphth

A female patient aged 51 years presented for a routine ophthalmic examination. She had a family history of ACG. The IOP was normal and gonioscopy revealed narrow angles. A double hump sign was seen on indentation gonioscopy. Slit-lamp examination showed a normal anterior chamber depth with flat iris plane. Ultrasound biomicroscopy (UBM) revealed anterior insertion of the iris root.

The case was discussed with the patient and a laser peripheral iridotomy was advised. The patient understood that laser peripheral iridotomy would not change the anatomy of her eye and, therefore, an acute attack could still happen.

The second choice was an argon laser peripheral iridoplasty, but an additional miotic may still be needed in the future to prevent the peripheral iris tissue from occluding the angle. Surgical pupilloplasty was then recommended to the patient along with cataract extraction due to nuclear sclerosis (Figures 7-10 and 7-11 and Video 7-2). Postoperative gonioscopy revealed open angles and periodic follow-ups were advised.

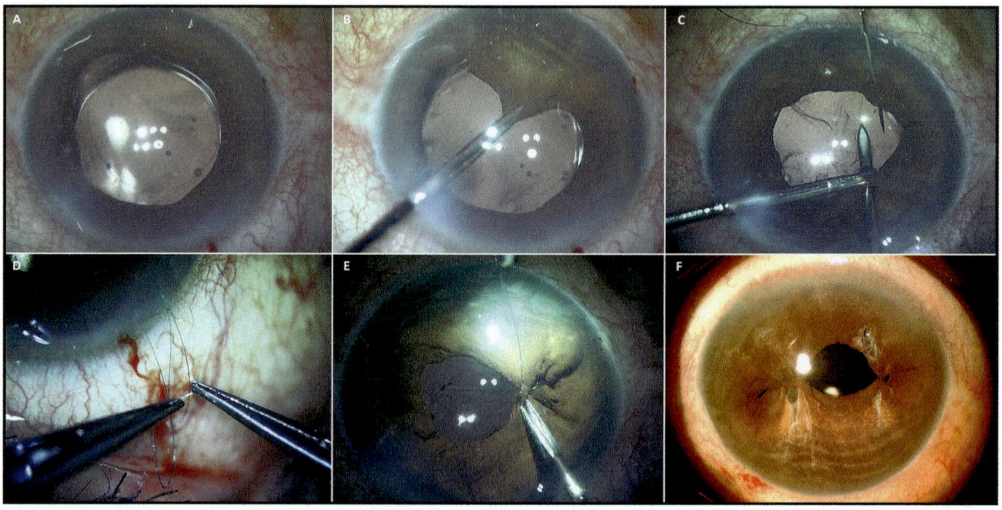

Figure 7-10. Clinical demonstration of SFT pupilloplasty in a case of plateau iris syndrome. (A) Lens removal and implantation of a foldable IOL. (B) The pupillary margin is held with end-opening forceps and pupillary stretching is performed. (C) A 10-0 suture on a long-armed needle is passed through the proximal iris tissue and a 26-gauge needle is introduced from the opposite paracentesis incision and is then passed through the distal iris tissue that is to be apposed. (D) The suture loop is withdrawn from the anterior chamber and the suture end is passed through the loop 4 times. (E) Both suture ends are pulled and the knot is cut with microscissors. (F) Intraoperative image after completion of SFT in 2 quadrants.

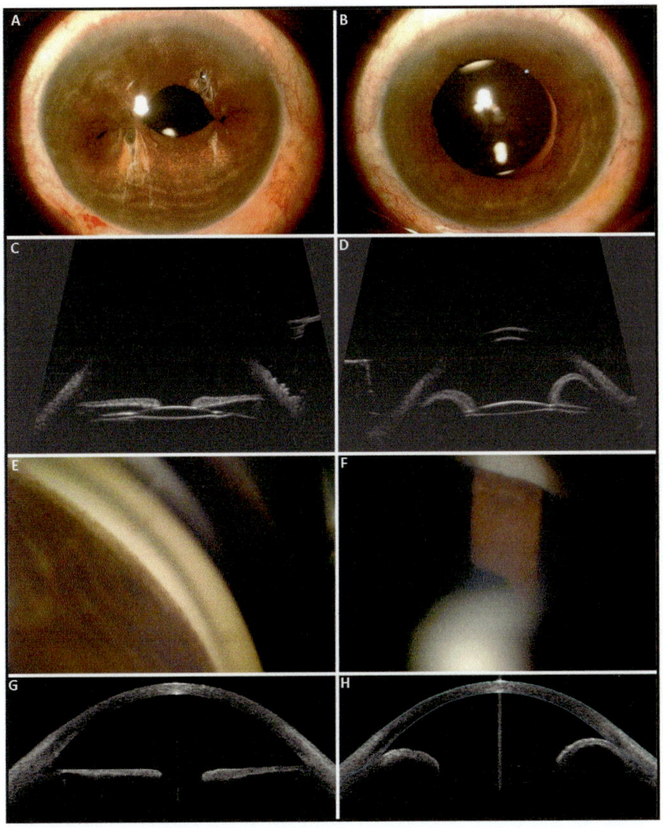

Figure 7-11. Comparative images of both eyes in a case of ACG with plateau iris syndrome and cataract extraction (left column: left eye with SFT; right column: right eye with no SFT). (A) Postoperative image of left eye with SFT and cataract extraction. (B) Postoperative image of right eye with only cataract extraction done. (C) UBM denotes open angles with flat iris tissue. (D) UBM denotes iris bombe with PAS. (E) Gonioscopy shows open angles. (F) Gonioscopy shows closed angles. (G) AS-OCT shows open angles. (H) AS-OCT shows angle closure with iris bombe.

References

1. Urrets-Zavalia A Jr. Fixed, dilated pupil, iris atrophy and secondary glaucoma. *Am J Ophthalmol.* 1963;56(8):257–265.
2. Jain R, Assi A, Murdoch IE. Urrets-Zavalia syndrome following trabeculectomy. *Br J Ophthalmol.* 2000;84(3):338-339.
3. Espana E, Ioannidis A, Tello C, Leibman JM, Foster P, Ritch R. Urrets-Zavalia syndrome as a complication of argon laser peripheral iridoplasty. *Br J Ophthalmol.* 2007;91(4):427–429.
4. Yuzbasioglu E, Helvacioglu F, Sencan S. Fixed, dilated pupil after phakic intraocular lens implantation. *J Cataract Refract Surg.* 2006;32(1):174–176.
5. Park SH, Kim SY, Kim HI, et al. Urrets-Zavalia syndrome following iris-claw phakic intraocular lens implantation. *J Refract Surg.* 2008;24(9):959-961.
6. Pérez-Cambrodí RJ, Piñero-Llorens DP, Ruiz-Fortes JP, Blanes-Mompó FJ, Cerviño-Expósito A. Fixed mydriatic pupil associated with an intraocular pressure rise as a complication of the implant of a phakic refractive lens (PRL). *Semin Ophthalmol.* 2014;29(4):205-209.
7. Maurino V, Allan BD, Stevens JD, et al. Fixed dilated pupil (Urrets-Zavalia syndrome) after air/gas injection after deep lamellar keratoplasty for keratoconus. *Am J Ophthalmol.* 2002;133(2):266-268.
8. Minasian M, Ayliffe W. Fixed dilated pupil following deep lamellar keratoplasty (Urrets-Zavalia syndrome). *Br J Ophthalmol.* 2002;86(1):115-116.
9. Maurino V, Allan BDS, Stevens JD, Tuft SJ. Fixed dilated pupil (Urrets-Zavalia syndrome) after air/gas injection after deep lamellar keratoplasty for keratoconus. *Am J Ophthalmol.* 2002;133(2):266-268.
10. Bozkurt KT, Acar BE, Acar S. Fixed dilated pupilla as a common complication of deep anterior lamellar keratoplasty complicated with Descemet membrane perforation. *Eur J Ophthalmol.* 2013;23(2):164-170.
11. Anwar DS, Chu CY, Prasher P, et al. Features of Urrets-Zavalia syndrome after Descemet stripping automated endothelial keratoplasty. *Cornea.* 2012;31(11):1330-1334.
12. Fournié P, Ponchel C, Malecaze F, et al. Fixed dilated pupil (Urrets-Zavalia syndrome) and anterior subcapsular cataract formation after Descemet stripping endothelial keratoplasty. *Cornea.* 2009;28(10):1184-1186.
13. Russell HC, Srinivasan S. Urrets-Zavalia syndrome following Descemet's stripping endothelial keratoplasty triple procedure. *Clin Experiment Ophthalmol.* 2011;39(1):85-87.
14. Chelnis JG, Sieminski SF, Reynolds JD. Urrets-Zavalia syndrome following goniotomy in a child. *JAAPOS.* 2012;16(3):312-313.
15. Aralikatti AK, Tomlins PJ, Shah S. Urrets-Zavalia syndrome following intracameral C3F8 injection for acute corneal hydrops. *Clin Experiment Ophthalmol.* 2008;36(2):198-199.
16. Narang P, Agarwal A. Single pass four-throw (SFT) pupilloplasty for Urrets-Zavalia syndrome. *Eur J Ophthalmol.* 2018;28(5):552-558.
17. Narang P, Agarwal A, Agarwal A. Silicon oil single-pass four-throw pupilloplasty for secondary angle-closure glaucoma associated with silicon oil tamponade. *Eur J Ophthalmol.* 2019;29(5):561-565.
18. Narang P, Agarwal A. Single-pass four-throw technique for pupilloplasty. *Eur J Ophthalmol.* 2017;27(4):506-508.
19. Narang P, Agarwal A, Kumar DA. Single pass four-throw pupilloplasty (SFT) for angle closure glaucoma. *Indian J Ophthalmol.* Article in Press.

Please visit www.routledge.com/9781630917265

to access additional material.

8

Pupilloplasty in Compartmentalizing the Eye
Endothelial Keratoplasty Including Pre-Descemet's Endothelial Keratoplasty With Glued Intraocular Lens/Yamane Technique

Amar Agarwal, MS, FRCS, FRCOphth, and Priya Narang, MS

Keywords

anterior chamber maintainer, Descemet's membrane endothelial keratoplasty, glued intraocular lens, pre-Descemet's endothelial keratoplasty, pupilloplasty, single-pass four-throw pupilloplasty, trocar anterior chamber maintainer, trocar, Yamane technique

The pupil in a human eye acts like a diaphragm that helps to filter the amount of light rays entering the eye. In the absence of the crystalline lens or the posterior capsule, the pupil forms an anatomical barrier between the anterior and posterior chamber. The importance of this barrier cannot be undermined in cases undergoing endothelial keratoplasty, especially when a secondary intraocular lens (IOL) fixation procedure has been performed (Videos 8-1 to 8-4).

Glued Intraocular Lens/Yamane Technique

Glued IOL was introduced in 2007 by Agarwal et al[1] as a technique for sutureless scleral fixation of the IOL via transscleral haptic tuck in patients with absent or deficient capsular support. In 2006, Scharioth Gabor first introduced the concept of intrascleral haptic fixation. This may be done as a primary procedure during cataract extraction in cases of posterior capsular rupture or as a secondary procedure in an aphakic patient. It may also be used for closed chamber translocation of a malpositioned or subluxated 3-piece IOL. However, many of the patients who need primary or secondary glued IOL implantation have already undergone complicated cataract surgery during which an IOL could not be implanted in the bag. Therefore, the chances of endothelial damage and the consequent need for a keratoplasty is higher in these patients. Depending on the severity of

Agarwal A, Agarwal A, eds. *Mastering Iris Repair: A Video Textbook of Iris Repair and Pupilloplasty Techniques* (pp 71-86).

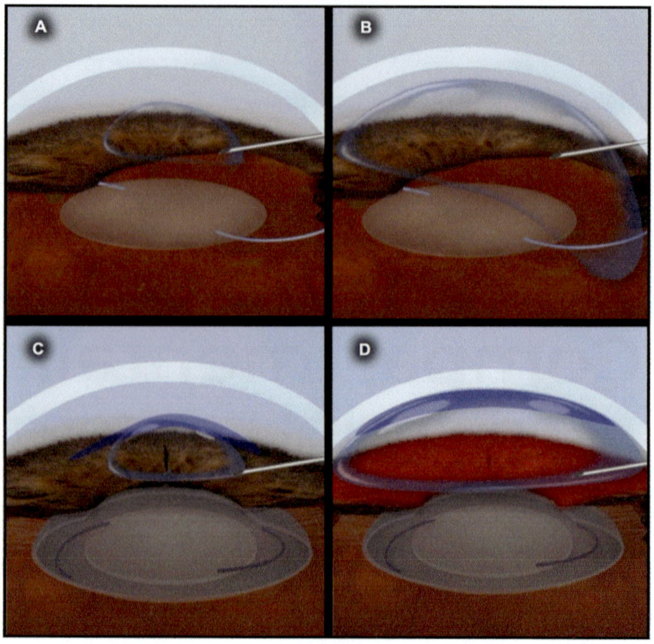

Figure 8-1. Illustration describing the role of pupilloplasty for achieving effective air tamponade. (A) Air being injected inside the anterior chamber. (B) Air seeps back into the vitreous cavity from the area of pupillary and iris defect. (C) Air being injected after pupilloplasty. (D) Effective air tamponade is achieved. (Republished with permission of Elsevier, from Narang P, Agarwal A. Triple procedure for pseudophakic bullous keratopathy in complicated cataract surgery: Glued IOL with single-pass four-throw pupilloplasty with pre-Descemet's endothelial keratoplasty. *J Cataract Refract Surg,* 45[4];2019; permission conveyed through Copyright Clearance Center, Inc.)

endothelial damage and corneal scarring, the patient may require either a penetrating or endothelial keratoplasty. Shin Yamane modified the intrascleral haptic fixation surgery, with the description of a "double-needle technique" that is popularly known as *Yamane's method*.[2]

Single-Pass Four-Throw Pupilloplasty in Endothelial Keratoplasty

The endothelial keratoplasty procedure involves the supplantation of the endothelial cell layer along with the Descemet's membrane that may or may not be supported with the layer of stroma in the donor graft. During endothelial keratoplasty, it is to prevent and minimize the loss of endothelial cells during the process of donor tissue preparation and also while inserting and repositioning the graft in the anterior chamber. The pupilloplasty procedure is often performed to prevent the escape of air into the vitreous cavity, to maintain the effective air tamponade in the anterior chamber, and to prevent the posterior dislocation of graft (Figure 8-1).[3-5] The technical manipulation of graft unfolding is mainly performed in the central portion of the anterior chamber where the knots of the pupilloplasty procedure are present. For this reason, Schoenberg and Price[6] presented a pupilloplasty technique in cases of endothelial keratoplasty with the knot directed toward the posterior of the iris tissue to prevent the mechanical rubbing of the knot with the donor graft.

The single-pass four-throw (SFT) pupilloplasty technique is very well described in a peer-reviewed paper,[7] and the authors perform it in cases that undergo pre-Descemet's endothelial keratoplasty (PDEK; Figure 8-2).[8,9] The SFT technique does not include a true knot formation. It involves an approximation loop with no securing loop that forms a helical structure, which is self-retaining and has a self-locking mechanism. A slight variation of the SFT technique is used where only one paracentesis incision is framed for the introduction of a 26-gauge needle to dock the 10-0 needle that has the suture attached to it. This has 2 potential advantages: it prevents the engagement and involvement of the 10-0 needle in the corneal bite, and the air tamponade can be more effective because the potential air leakage is decreased due to only one paracentesis incision. The paracentesis incision should be carefully placed depending on the site of iris defect and the ease of maneuverability. Moreover, the loop withdrawal is performed from the paracentesis side as only 1 paracentesis incision is framed (see Video 8-1).

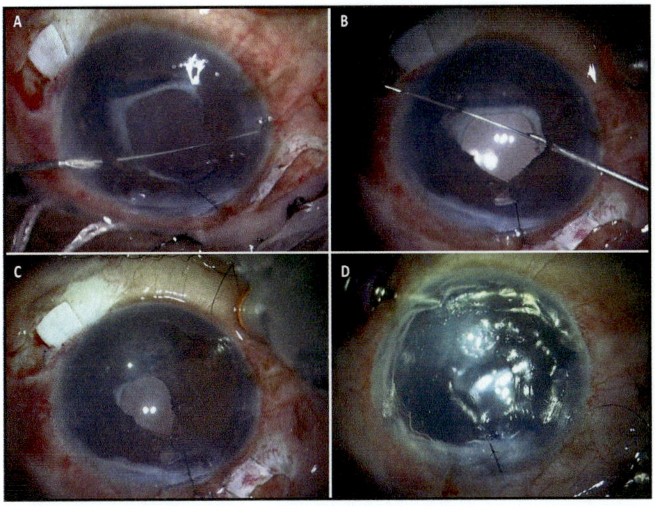

Figure 8-2. SFT for PDEK. (A) A 10-0 suture attached to the long arm of the needle is passed through the corneal tissue and a 26-gauge needle is introduced from the opposite side through the paracentesis incision. The 10-0 needle is docked into the barrel of 26-gauge needle, and SFT is performed. (B) SFT being performed on the opposite side. (C) Pupil reconstruction completed. (D) Graft reposition in PDEK procedure with air fill in anterior chamber.

When trimmed, the suture ends are essentially parallel to the surface of the iris and do not protrude into the anterior chamber. Hence, the chances of the knot rubbing on to the endothelial cells of the donor graft are negligible. In a study conducted by the authors, anterior segment optical coherence tomography (AS-OCT) analysis was done with the images being taken at the level of iris that demonstrated an elevation of around 136 to 160 µm in the longitudinal meridian and 160 to 175 µm in the cross-sectional meridian from the adjoining iris plane.[10] The SFT procedure causes virtually no damage from the knot of the suture that potentially lies parallel to the iris tissue and, therefore, has a definite role in cases undergoing endothelial keratoplasty.

SFT with PDEK in failed grafts with penetrating keratoplasty has been shown to yield favorable outcomes (Figure 8-3). These are often Urrets-Zavalia syndrome cases that respond well to surgical pupilloplasty, which results in a lowering of intraocular pressure.[11] It has the added advantage of enhancing the visual potential in cases undergoing endothelial keratoplasty. The combined procedure of SFT with PDEK and the triple procedure of SFT with PDEK and glued IOL[12] (Figures 8-4 through 8-6) have been documented to provide good visual outcomes, thereby optimizing the suboptimal outcomes from the prior surgery.

Principles of Combining Glued Intraocular Lens With Endothelial Keratoplasty

In aphakic eyes, a loss of bicamerality of the eye occurs that leads to posterior migration of the air bubble used for attaching the endothelial keratoplasty graft. This increases the risk for a postoperative partial or total graft detachment, forward bowing of the iris, iris-graft touch, and graft dislocation into the vitreous, all of which can necessitate secondary procedures, such as refloating, rebubbling, vitrectomy, and anterior chamber formation, and increase graft endothelial cell loss. An effective compartmentalization of the eye can be achieved through the glued IOL technique. The advantages of glued IOL are posterior chamber placement of the IOL with ease of centration, scleral fixation, and stable and sturdy fixation without pseudophakodonesis. It is our preferred technique when combining with endothelial keratoplasty. In contrast, anterior chamber IOLs have the disadvantage of decreased anterior chamber space, iris fixated IOLs require an intact iris all around, and sutured scleral fixated IOLs have a greater risk of pseudophakodonesis and greater difficulty in centration (Figures 8-7 through 8-9 and Video 8-2).

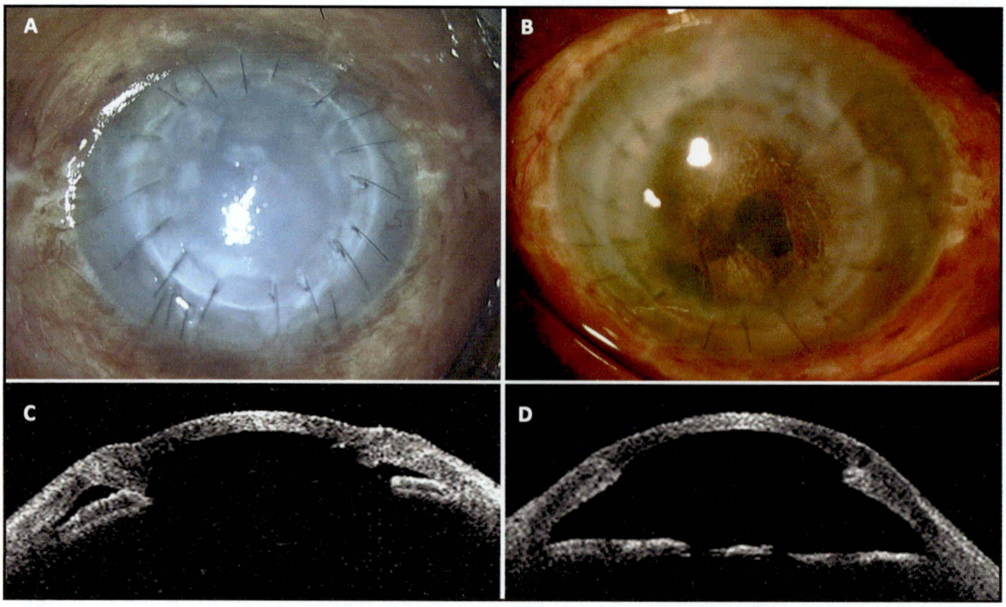

Figure 8-3. SFT with PDEK in failed penetrating keratoplasty. (A) Failed penetrating keratoplasty graft. (B) Postoperative image following SFT with PDEK. (C) Preoperative AS-OCT image. (D) Postoperative AS-OCT image demonstrating pupil reconstruction with decreased thickness of cornea due to resolution of edema.

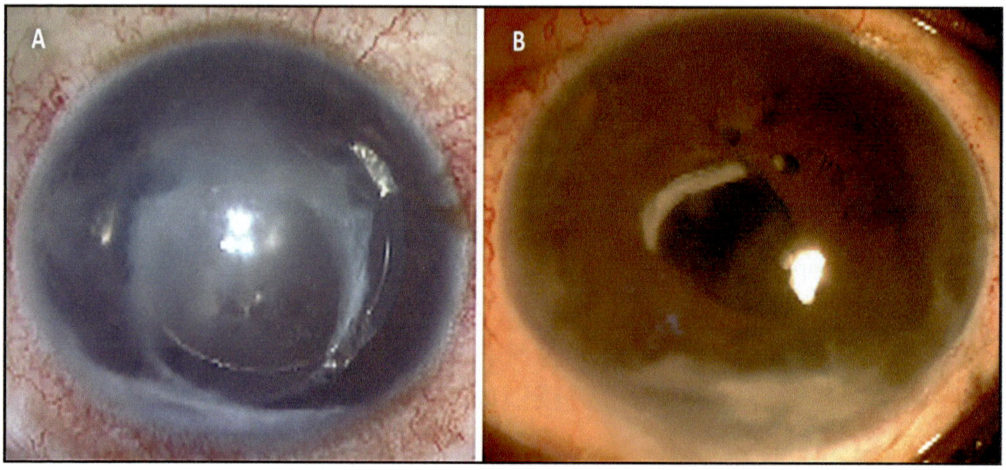

Figure 8-4. SFT with PDEK in pseudophakic bullous keratopathy. (A) Preoperative image of a case with anterior chamber IOL. (B) Postoperative image with clear graft and SFT procedure along with anterior chamber IOL explantation and glued IOL procedure.

The procedure is started as a conventional glued IOL. An anterior chamber maintainer (ACM) or a trocar anterior chamber maintainer (TACM) is inserted. Conjunctival flaps and lamellar scleral flaps are then made 180 degrees apart as explained earlier followed by 20/22-gauge sclerotomies under the scleral flap about 1 mm from the limbus. This is followed by limited 23-gauge vitrectomy through the sclerotomies followed by glued IOL implantation. The haptics are tucked in the Scharioth pockets, and the flaps may be glued down. As the posterior capsule is unlikely to be intact, there is still a chance of posterior migration of air that is injected into the anterior chamber for graft support. Migration of air behind the IOL leads to insufficient support for the graft with consequent graft detachment. It is, therefore, imperative to have a good iris diaphragm IOL separating the anterior chamber from the vitreous cavity. Therefore, when combining a glued IOL with endothelial keratoplasty, the sclerotomy should be made slightly closer to the limbus

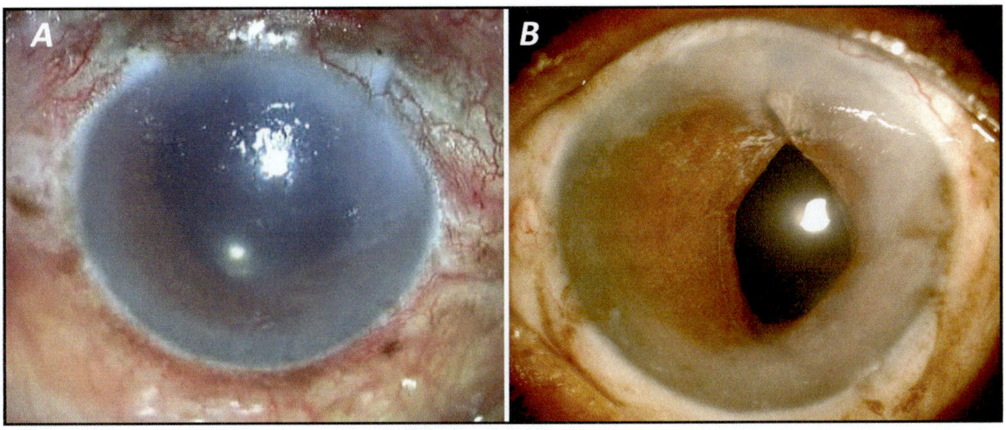

Figure 8-5. Clinical images of cases with pseudophakic bullous keratopathy. (A) Preoperative image of cases with pseudophakic bullous keratopathy. (B) Postoperative images of cases that underwent triple procedures.

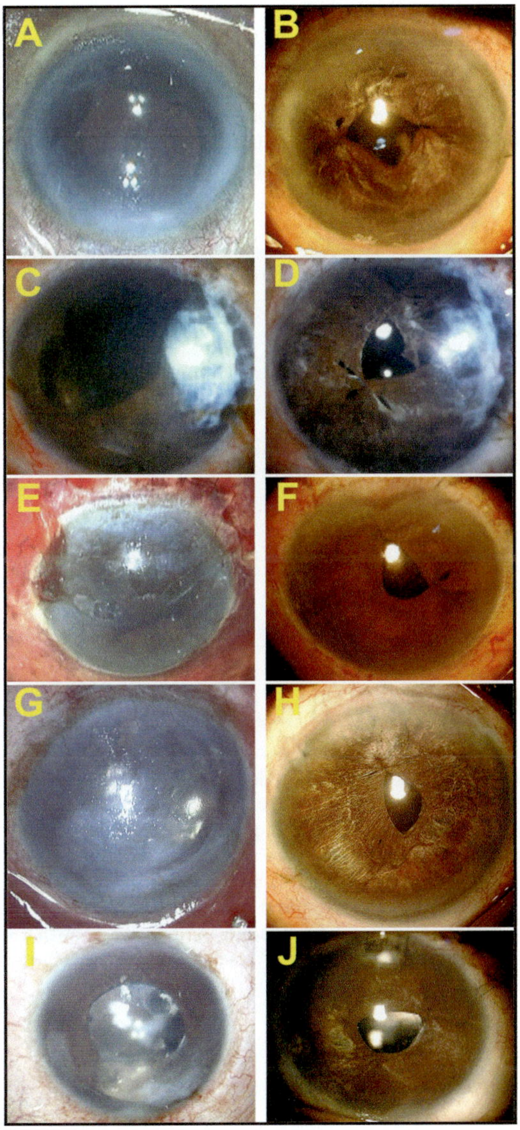

Figure 8-6. (A, C, E, G, I) Preoperative images of cases and (B, D, F, H, J) postoperative images of the same cases. (Republished with permission of Elsevier, from Narang P, Agarwal A. Triple procedure for pseudophakic bullous keratopathy in complicated cataract surgery: Glued IOL with single-pass four-throw pupilloplasty with pre-Descemet's endothelial keratoplasty. *J Cataract Refract Surg*, 45[4];2019; permission conveyed through Copyright Clearance Center, Inc.)

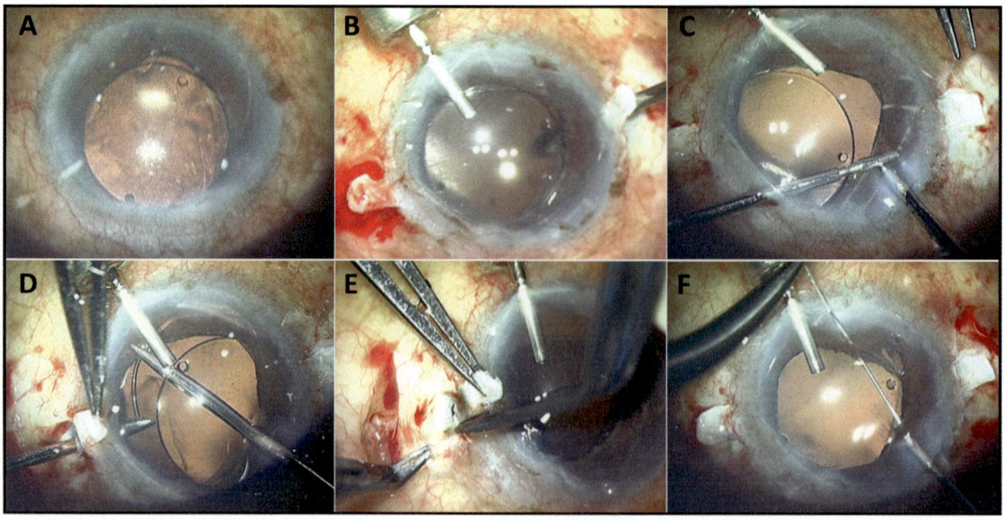

Figure 8-7. Part 1: PDEK with glued IOL. (A) Pseudophakic bullous keratopathy. Note the corneal haze and a single-piece non-foldable posterior chamber IOL in the anterior chamber. (B) ACM fixed. One can also fix a TACM or a trocar cannula in the pars plana. Two sclera flaps created 180 degrees apart and a 20/22-gauge sclerotomy created with a needle 1 mm from the limbus. (C) After vitrectomy, the haptics are grasped with glued IOL forceps and externalized using the handshake technique. (D) One should be careful when externalizing the haptics as this is a single-piece non-foldable IOL. If haptics break, then the IOL can be explanted and replaced with a 3-piece IOL. (E) Scharioth pocket created with a 26-gauge needle and haptics tucked in them. (F) Pupilloplasty completed.

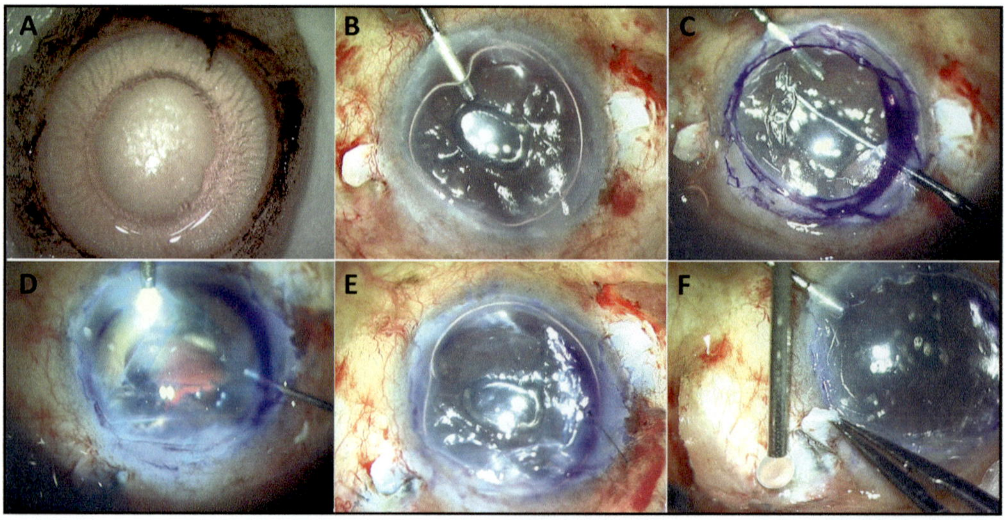

Figure 8-8. Part 2: PDEK with glued IOL. (A) Type 1 big bubble created. One can do the PDEK and glued IOL at the same time, but 2 steps are preferred so that the glued IOL heals before PDEK is performed 1 month later. Another advantage is that, because donor corneas are not readily available, the glued IOL can be performed while waiting for a donor cornea. (B) Air pump-assisted PDEK. In this case, the air pump is connected to the TACM or ACM so that air is continuously flowing inside the anterior chamber. If one is doing PDEK with glued IOL in one sitting, it is better to have a trocar cannula in the pars plana with fluid being passed inside and an ACM or a TACM in the anterior chamber passing air. This way hypotony will be avoided and one can control the amount of fluid being passed inside the eye. (C) Descemetorhexis. (D) PDEK graft injected inside the anterior chamber and unrolled with the help of an endoilluminator. (E) Graft attached. (F) Glue applied.

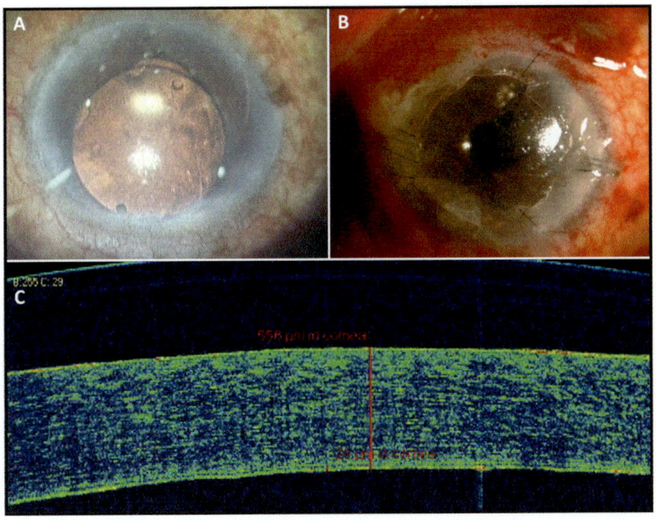

Figure 8-9. Part 3: PDEK with glued IOL. (A) Preoperative. (B) Postoperative day 1. (C) AS-OCT shows an attached graft.

than usual in order to decrease the potential gap between the iris and the IOL. At the same time, an iridoplasty should be performed to obtain a round pupil that overlaps the IOL optic all around. Once this is done, the adequacy of air fill is checked by turning off the infusion and checking the air fill. If inadequate, the pupil may need to become smaller or the IOL may need to come closer to the iris. A well-formed iris diaphragm IOL prevents air from going back into the vitreous cavity and allows good postoperative support for the graft. Once the air fill is found to be adequate, air is attached to the ACM through an air pump and host descemetorhexis is performed. The endothelial keratoplasty graft is then injected into the anterior chamber, unfolded, and floated up using air. In cases with subluxated or dislocated 3-piece IOL needing endothelial keratoplasty, a closed chamber translocation of the subluxated IOL into a glued IOL may be done using the handshake technique. This is followed by iridoplasty, if required, and endothelial keratoplasty (see Video 8-3).

Cases with malpositioned single-piece IOL or anterior chamber IOL need an enlargement of the wound followed by explantation of the IOL. This is followed by the technique described previously. Construction of a scleral tunnel for IOL explantation or a 3-mm L-shaped scleral tunnel incision gives very good wound closure and excellent anterior chamber stability.

A potential complication of combining glued IOL with endothelial keratoplasty is the risk for hypotony and subsequent graft detachment in the postoperative period. Hypotony can lead to detachment of the endothelial keratoplasty graft simply from the eyelids pushing on the cornea with normal eyelid movements. This risk can be decreased by ensuring that the globe is adequately pressurized at the end of surgery. As noted, this is done by achieving an adequately tight air bubble in the anterior chamber. If the globe still feels hypotonic, air is injected through the pars plicata into the vitreous cavity with a 30-gauge needle under direct visualization of the needle tip in the vitreous cavity. At the conclusion of surgery, the surgeon should make sure that the sclerotomies are well sealed by the scleral flaps using fibrin glue. All corneal incisions can also be sealed using fibrin glue to avoid any postoperative leak of aqueous or escape of air that could increase the risk of detachment. Postoperatively, patients should be monitored closely to look for any evidence of partial or total graft detachments and taken for rebubbling if required.

A properly positioned IOL and a successful iridoplasty decrease the chances of the graft slipping into the vitreous cavity during surgery. However, this possibility should be kept in mind and care should be taken to avoid any inappropriate fluidics that may cause a graft drop.

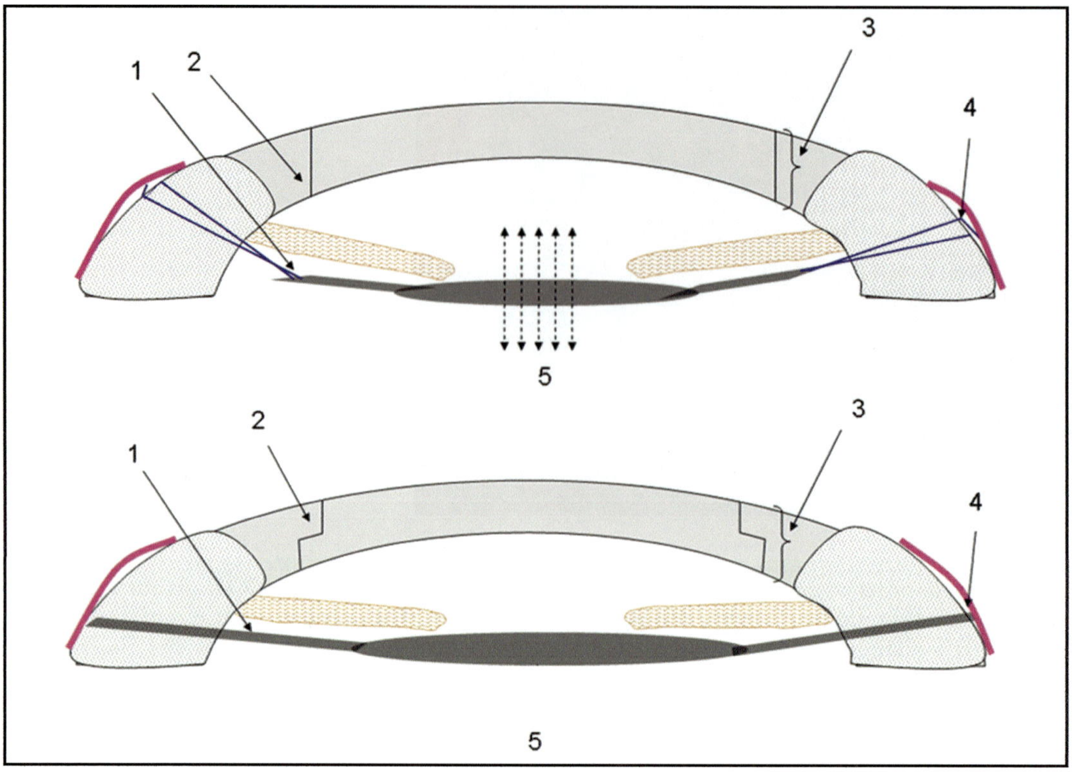

Figure 8-10. Diagram showing biomechanical and kinetic properties of manual keratoplasty with transscleral suture-fixated posterior chamber IOL (top) and femtosecond-assisted keratoplasty with glued IOL (bottom). Differences between the 2 approaches are indicated by the numbers. (1, top) Haptic–suture junction in the transscleral suture-fixated IOL, with the IOL hanging like a hammock. (1, bottom) Rigid polymethyl methacrylate haptic in glued IOL fixated with the sclera. (2, top) Transverse graft–host junction. (2, bottom) More stable top-hat configuration. (3, top) Size of epithelial side (outer cut) same as that of endothelial side (inner cut). (3, bottom) Size of epithelial side (outer cut) less than that of endothelial side (inner cut), leading to greater number of endothelial cells for smaller epithelial load and placement of sutures farther from limbus. (4, top) Knots in transscleral suture-fixated IOL may degrade and slip. (4, bottom) Haptic is securely tucked and sealed with fibrin glue in glued IOL. (5, top) More pseudophacodonesis with transscleral suture-fixated IOL. (5, bottom) Less pseudophacodonesis with glued IOL. (Republished with permission of Elsevier, from Prakash G, Jacob S, Ashok Kumar D, Narsimhan S, Agarwal A, Agarwal A. Femtosecond-assisted keratoplasty with fibrin glue-assisted sutureless posterior chamber lens implantation: new triple procedure. *J Cataract Refract Surg*, 35[6];2009; permission conveyed through Copyright Clearance Center, Inc.)

Advantages

The glued IOL technique can be performed with less open-sky time compared to other secondary IOL fixation techniques. Once the haptics have been exteriorized, the optic acts as a tamponade and is helpful in preventing expulsive hemorrhage (Figure 8-10). It can also be done with any 3-piece IOL available. There is no need for a special IOL with eyelets on the haptic. The glued IOL technique may be performed in hypotonous eyes with centration adjusted after the graft is sutured and the globe is formed. Lack of pseudophacodonesis is another advantage in the glued IOL technique compared to other secondary IOL fixation techniques (Figures 8-11 through 8-13).

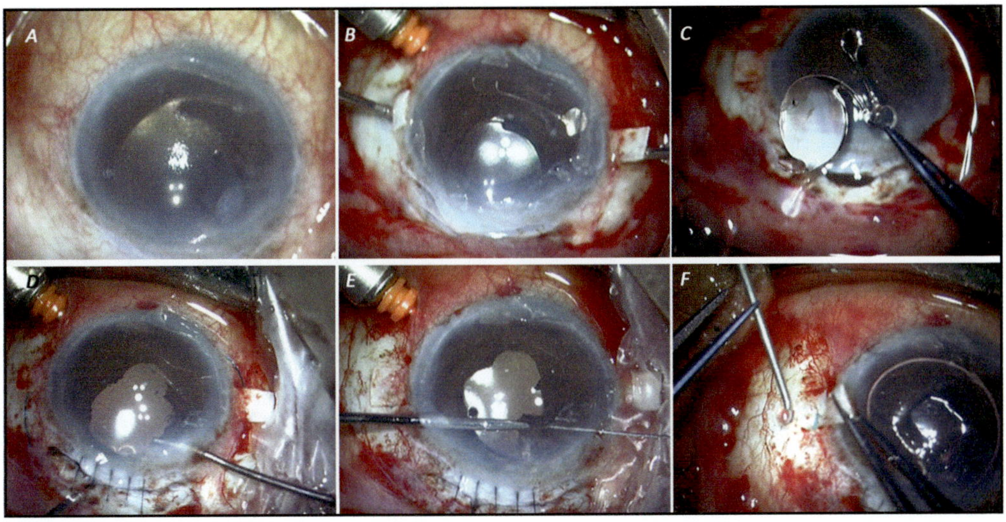

Figure 8-11. Part 1: PDEK with glued IOL. (A) Pseudophakic bullous keratopathy. Note the corneal haze and an anterior chamber IOL in the eye. (B) Trocar cannula fixed. Two sclera flaps created 180 degrees apart and a 20/22-gauge sclerotomy created with a needle 1 mm from the limbus. (C) After vitrectomy, the haptics are grasped with glued IOL forceps and the anterior chamber IOL explanted. (D) Glued IOL in place. Note the haptics externalized under the scleral flaps. Suturing of the scleral tunnel is completed. (E) SFT pupilloplasty performed to make the pupil smaller so that air remains in the anterior chamber and does not go into the vitreous cavity when PDEK is performed. (F) Fibrin glue applied.

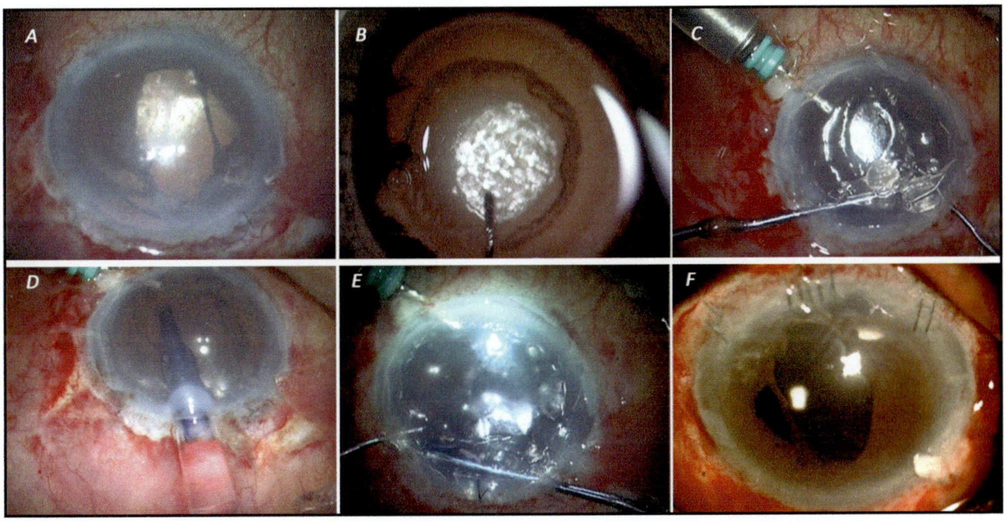

Figure 8-12. Part 2: PDEK with glued IOL. (A) One month after glued IOL. Note the corneal haze. (B) Type 1 big bubble created. One can do the PDEK and glued IOL at the same time, but 2 steps are preferred so that the glued IOL heals before PDEK is performed 1 month later. Another advantage is that donor corneas are not readily available so the glued IOL can be performed while waiting for a donor cornea. (C) Descemetorhexis being performed. Air pump–assisted PDEK. In this procedure, the air pump is connected to the TACM or ACM so that air is continuously flowing inside the anterior chamber. If one is doing PDEK with glued IOL in one sitting it is better to have a trocar cannula in the pars plana with fluid being passed inside and an ACM or TACM in the anterior chamber passing air. This way there will not be any hypotony and one can control the amount of fluid being passed inside the eye. (D) PDEK graft injected inside the anterior chamber. (E) PDEK graft unrolled with the help of an endoilluminator. (F) Postoperative week 1.

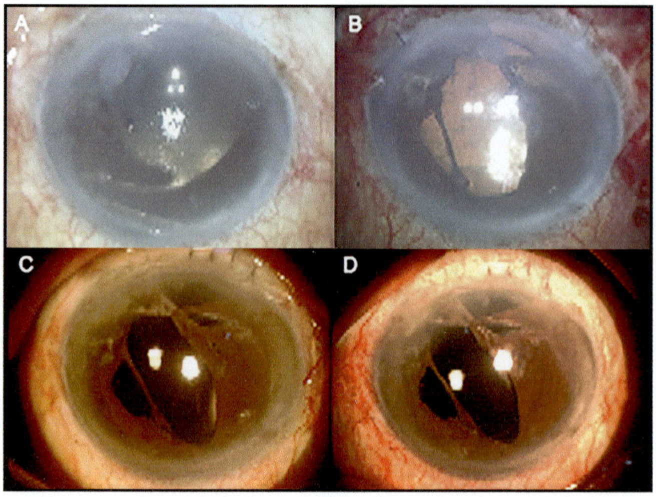

Figure 8-13. Part 3: PDEK with glued IOL. (A) Preoperative. (B) One month following glued IOL. (C) Two months following PDEK, vision 6/12. (D) Four months following PDEK, vision 6/6.

CASE PRESENTATION 1

TRIPLE PROCEDURE OF PRE-DESCEMET'S ENDOTHELIAL KERATOPLASTY WITH GLUED INTRAOCULAR LENS AND SINGLE-PASS FOUR-THROW PUPILLOPLASTY

Amar Agarwal, MS, FRCS, FRCOphth and Priya Narang, MS

A patient with 1 eye presented with history of dimness of vision (20/200 on Snellen's chart) since he got operated for cataract surgery almost 1 year ago. Slit-lamp examination revealed a scarred cornea that completely impaired the visualization of intraocular structures. A retro-corneal fibrotic membrane was present that was adhered to the iris tissue. Ultrasound biomicroscopy revealed decentration of the IOL. An endothelial keratoplasty procedure was planned along with management of secondary IOL fixation. Informed consent was taken after proper counselling of the patient.

The case was managed with removal of fibrotic membrane followed by refixation of the 3-piece IOL that was present inside the eye with the glued IOL procedure. SFT pupilloplasty was performed that helped to compartmentalize the eye followed by PDEK (Figures 8-14 through 8-17 and Video 8-5).

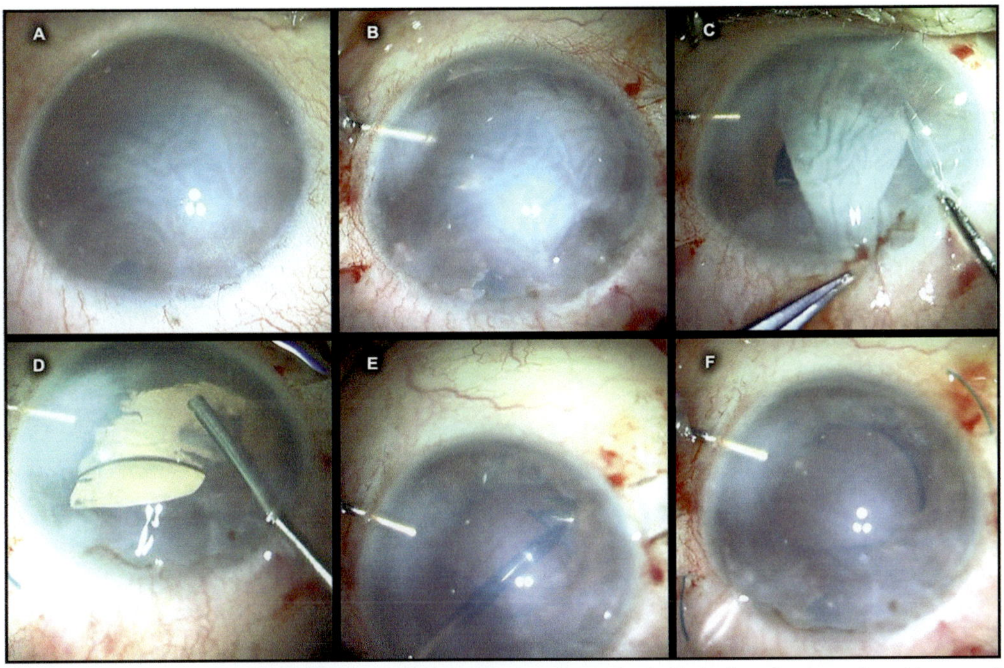

Figure 8-14. Surgical steps of triple procedure. (A) A case of pseudophakic bullous keratopathy with scarred cornea. (B) A TACM is placed in position and 2 partial-thickness scleral flaps are made 180 degrees opposite to each other. (C) The fibrotic-scarred tissue on the endothelial side is cut and removed. This enhances the intraoperative visualization. (D) A subluxated 3-piece IOL is visualized. Limited anterior vitrectomy is performed. (E) Handshake technique is performed for trailing haptic externalization. (F) Both the haptics are externalized. (Republished with permission of Elsevier, from Narang P, Agarwal A. Triple procedure for pseudophakic bullous keratopathy in complicated cataract surgery: Glued IOL with single-pass four-throw pupilloplasty with pre-Descemet's endothelial keratoplasty. *J Cataract Refract Surg*, 45[4];2019; permission conveyed through Copyright Clearance Center, Inc.)

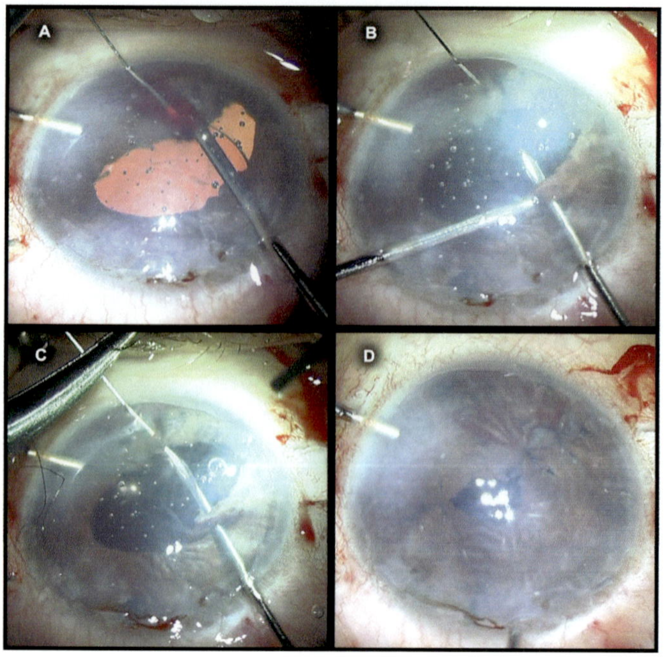

Figure 8-15. Surgical steps of triple procedure. (A) A 10-0 suture on a long-armed needle is passed through the paracentesis incision, and the proximal part of the iris tissue to be apposed is held. The needle is passed through it. (B) A 26-gauge needle is passed through the paracentesis incision from the opposite side. (C) The 10-0 needle is threaded into the barrel of a 26-gauge needle and the needle is withdrawn. A Sinskey hook is passed through the anterior chamber and the loop is withdrawn from the anterior chamber. The suture end is passed through the loop 4 times and both the suture ends are pulled. The knot slides inside the anterior chamber. (D) SFT is completed and the iris defects are closed.(Republished with permission of Elsevier, from Narang P, Agarwal A. Triple procedure for pseudophakic bullous keratopathy in complicated cataract surgery: Glued IOL with single-pass four-throw pupilloplasty with pre-Descemet's endothelial keratoplasty. *J Cataract Refract Surg*, 45[4];2019; permission conveyed through Copyright Clearance Center, Inc.)

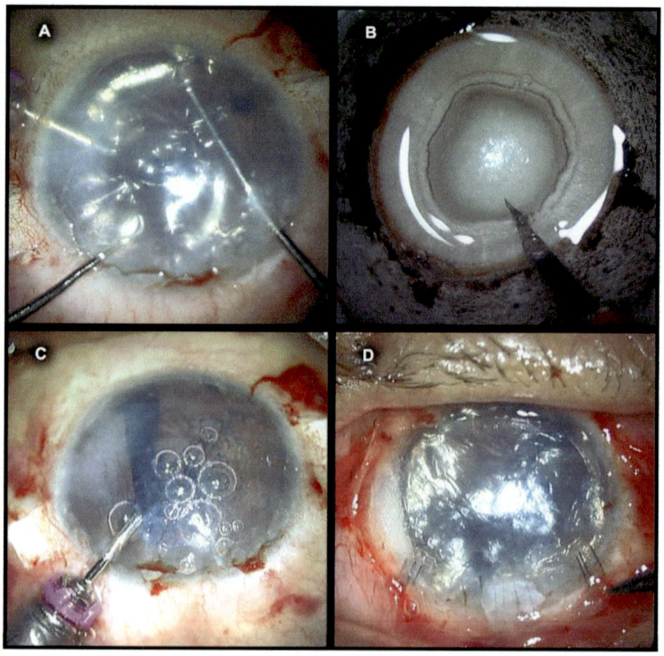

Figure 8-16. Surgical steps of triple procedure. (A) A reverse Sinskey hook is introduced and the descemetorhexis is completed. (B) A type 1 big bubble is created and the edge of the bubble is ruptured with side port blade. (C) The graft is loaded onto the cartridge of the foldable IOL and is injected inside the anterior chamber. (D) The graft is unrolled and air is injected beneath the graft to adhere it to the host bed. (Republished with permission of Elsevier, from Narang P, Agarwal A. Triple procedure for pseudophakic bullous keratopathy in complicated cataract surgery: Glued IOL with single-pass four-throw pupilloplasty with pre-Descemet's endothelial keratoplasty. *J Cataract Refract Surg*, 45[4];2019; permission conveyed through Copyright Clearance Center, Inc.)

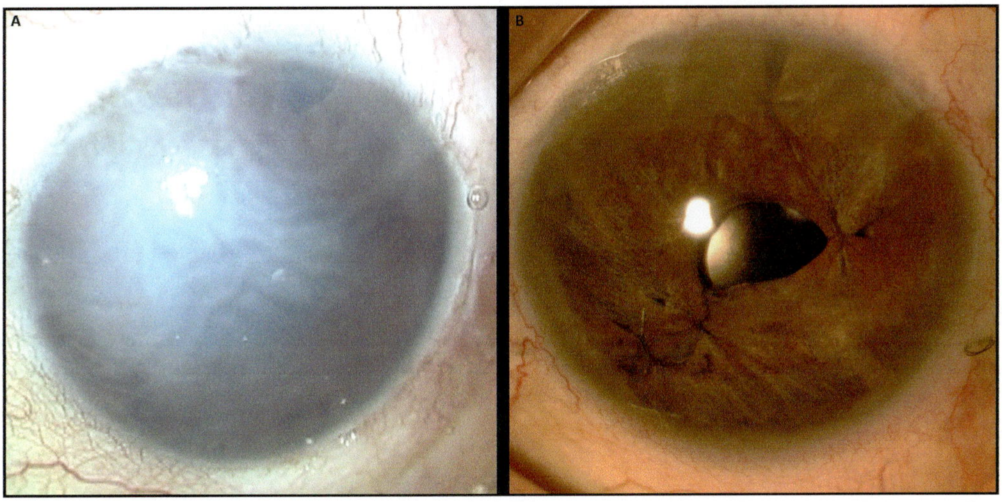

Figure 8-17. Clinical images. (A) Preoperative image of the case. (B) Postoperative image of the case after triple procedure.

Case Presentation 2

Yamane Technique. Flanged Intrascleral Intraocular Lens Fixation With Double-Needle Technique

Shin Yamane, MD, PhD

The intrascleral IOL fixation technique was described by Gabor and Pavlidis[13] and Agarwal et al[1] as a sutureless technique for IOL fixation. This technique has become a popular procedure because it has some advantages over conventional transscleral suturing of the IOL. Flanged IOL fixation is a new surgical procedure that can be carried out via the conjunctiva in which the haptics of the IOL are strongly fixed to the sclera without using suture or glue. This technique is simple but not easy. The surgeon needs to understand some key points of the technique (Videos 8-6 and 8-7).

Technique

- Pars plana vitrectomy or anterior vitrectomy.
- Subluxated crystalline lens or dislocated IOL removal.
- A 3-piece IOL insertion into the anterior chamber. The trailing haptic must be kept outside to prevent the IOL from falling into the vitreous cavity.
- Angled sclerotomies made with a 30-gauge thin wall needle through the conjunctiva 2 mm from the limbus
- Insertion of the leading haptic into the lumen of the needle using forceps.
- A second sclerotomy made with a 30-gauge thin-wall needle 180 degrees from the first sclerotomy.
- Insertion of the trailing haptic into the lumen of the second needle while the first needle is put on the conjunctiva
- Externalization of the haptics onto the conjunctiva with the needles.
- Cauterization of the ends of the haptics using an ophthalmic cautery device (Accu-Temp Cautery, Beaver-Visitec International) to make a flange with a diameter of 0.3 mm.
- Fixation of the flange of the haptics into the scleral tunnels.
- Peripheral iridotomy using the vitrectomy cutter after miosis.

Pearls of Surgery

- 30-gauge thin wall needle: The TSK Ultra Thin Wall Needle is available in Japan (Tochigi Seiko), the United States (Delasco Dermatologic Lab and Supply), and the Netherlands (TSK Laboratory Europe). The inner diameter of the needle must be 0.18 mm or more. The outer diameter of the needle should not be larger than the flange of the IOL haptics. A 27-gauge needle is available if the diameter of the flange is over 0.4 mm.
- The positional relationship of the wounds: The wound where the IOL is inserted and the site where the 30-gauge needle is inserted should be separated by approximately 90 degrees (Figure 8-18).
- Double-needle technique: Placing the leading haptic in the inner cavity of the 30-gauge needle makes the positional relationship of the trailing haptic and the second 30-gauge needle appropriate and facilitates easy insertion. If the leading haptic is pulled out together with the 30-gauge needle, the IOL will rotate counterclockwise. It is difficult to insert the tip of the trailing haptic into a 30-gauge needle in this situation (Figure 8-19).

- The insertion angle of the 30-gauge needle: In order to avoid IOL tilt and dislocation, the haptics must be fixed symmetrically. We have developed a device to stabilize the direction of the needles that will help fixate the IOL in the perfect position.
- Making and fixation of the flange: The cautery should not touch the haptic to avoid adhesion. The haptic should be dry to avoid twisted the flange. The appropriate length of the haptic to cauterize is 0.5 to 1.0 mm. If the size of the flange is too large to insert into the scleral tunnel, the entry site of the scleral tunnel should be enlarged using a 30-gauge needle.

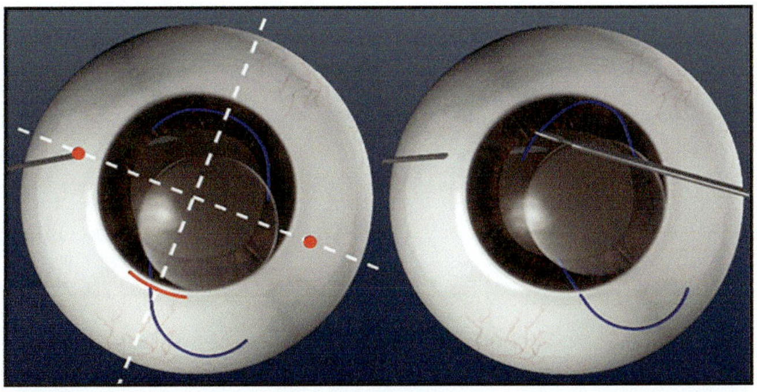

Figure 8-18. The positional relationship of the wounds. It is easy to insert the leading haptic into the needle if the positional relationship of the wounds is appropriate (left). If the wounds are too distant, the haptic hits the cornea (right).

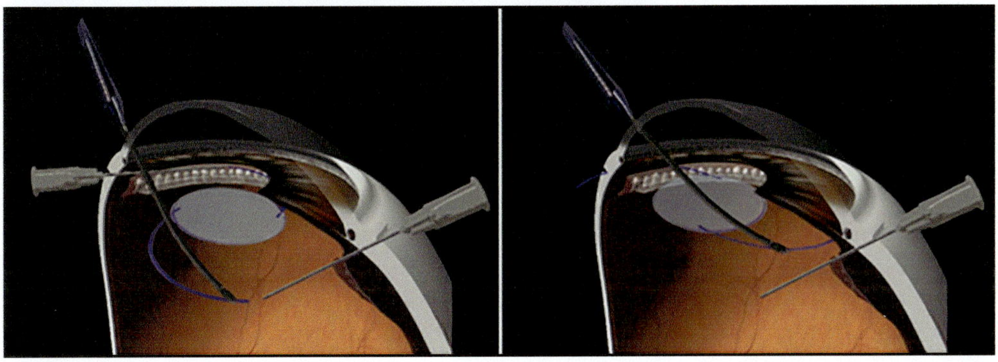

Figure 8-19. Double-needle technique. The correct position (left). The leading haptic is in the needle. It is difficult to insert the tip of the trailing haptic into a 30-gauge needle after pulling out of the leading haptic from the needle (right).

References

1. Agarwal A, Kumar DA, Jacob S, Baid C, Agarwal A, Srinivasan S. Fibrin glue–assisted sutureless posterior chamber intraocular lens implantation in eyes with deficient posterior capsules. *J Cataract Refract Surg.* 2008;34: 1433–1438.
2. Yamane S, Sato S, Maruyama-Inoue M, Kadonosono K. Flanged intrascleral intraocular lens fixation with double-needle technique. *Ophthalmology.* 2017;124:1136-1142.
3. Narang P, Agarwal A, Kumar DA. Single-pass 4-throw pupilloplasty for pre-Descemet endothelial keratoplasty. *Cornea.* 2017;36:1580-1583.
4. Narang P, Agarwal A, Dua HS, Kumar DA, Jacob S, Agarwal A. Glued intrascleral fixation of intraocular lens with pupilloplasty and pre-Descemet endothelial keratoplasty: a triple procedure. *Cornea.* 2015;34:1627-1631.
5. Agarwal A, Agarwal A, Narang P, Kumar DA, Jacob S. Pre-Descemet endothelial keratoplasty with infant donor corneas: a prospective analysis. *Cornea.* 2015;34:859-865.
6. Schoenberg ED, Price FW Jr. Modification of Siepser sliding suture technique for iris repair and endothelial keratoplasty. *J Cataract Refract Surg.* 2014;40:705-708.
7. Narang P, Agarwal A. Single-pass four-throw technique for pupilloplasty. *Eur J Ophthalmol.* 2017;27:506-508.
8. Agarwal A, Dua HS, Narang P et al. Pre-Descemet's endothelial keratoplasty (PDEK). *Br J Ophthalmol.* 2014;98:1181-1185.
9. Dua HS, Faraj LA, Said DG, et al. Human corneal anatomy redefined. A novel pre-Descemet's layer (Dua's layer). *Ophthalmology.* 2013;120:1778–1785.
10. Narang P, Agarwal A, Kumar DA. Single pass 4-throw pupilloplasty for pre-Descemet's endothelial keratoplasty. *Cornea.* 2017;36(12):1580-1583
11. Narang P, Agarwal A. Single pass four-throw pupilloplasty for Urrets-Zavalia syndrome. *Eur J Ophthalmol.* 2018;28(5):552-558.
12. Narang P, Agarwal A. Triple procedure for pseudophakic bullous keratopathy in complicated cataract surgery: glued IOL with single pass four-throw pupilloplasty with pre-Descemet's endothelial keratoplasty. *J Cataract Refract Surg.* 2019;45(4):398-403.
13. Gabor SG, Pavlidis MM. Sutureless intrascleral posterior chamber intraocular lens fixation. *J Cataract Refract Surg.* 2007;33:1851-1854.

Please visit www.routledge.com/9781630917265 to access additional material.

9

Iris Prosthesis Devices

David T. Truong MD and Kevin M. Miller, MD

Keywords

artificial iris, iridodialysis, iris defects, iris prosthesis, iris reconstruction, modified capsular tension rings, pupilloplasty

Patients with iris defects often suffer from poor cosmesis and debilitating visual dysfunction, including glare, photophobia, monocular diplopia, loss of visual acuity, and poor contrast sensitivity. Iris reconstruction[1-18] offers a means of addressing these problems when more conservative measures, such as darkly tinted sunglasses, colored or artificial pupil contact lenses, or corneal tattooing, are insufficient. Iris defects, both congenital and acquired, are often associated with significant ocular comorbidities that must be managed concurrently by the enterprising surgeon. Affected eyes have often had multiple surgeries prior to presentation, and the surgical approach depends upon the extent of iris defect and the overall condition of the eye including the cornea, iris, lens or capsular bag, and retina (Video 9-1).

Iris reconstruction techniques fall broadly into 2 categories: suture repair and prosthetic iris implantation. Suture repair can be effective for the repair of small iris lacerations or defects, iridodialyses, and abnormalities of the pupillary sphincter. When suture repair is inadequate, prosthetic iris implantation may be necessary to compensate for larger areas of lost stromal tissue.

Management of Large Iris Defects

Artificial iris device implantation is often the best approach for patients with significant iris stromal loss. Excluding cosmetic artificial iris devices, which have a high complication rate, there

Agarwal A, Agarwal A, eds. *Mastering Iris Repair: A Video Textbook of Iris Repair and Pupilloplasty Techniques* (pp 87-96).

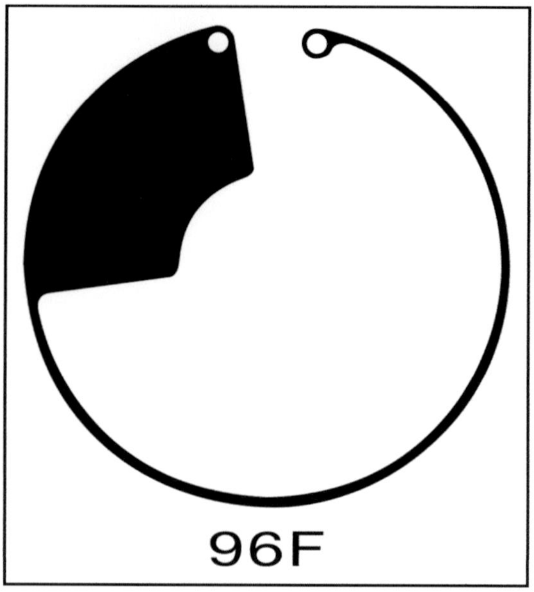

Figure 9-1. This 96F modified capsular tension ring (Morcher GmbH) contains a single black occluder paddle that subtends 90 degrees. (Reprinted with permission from Morcher GmbH.)

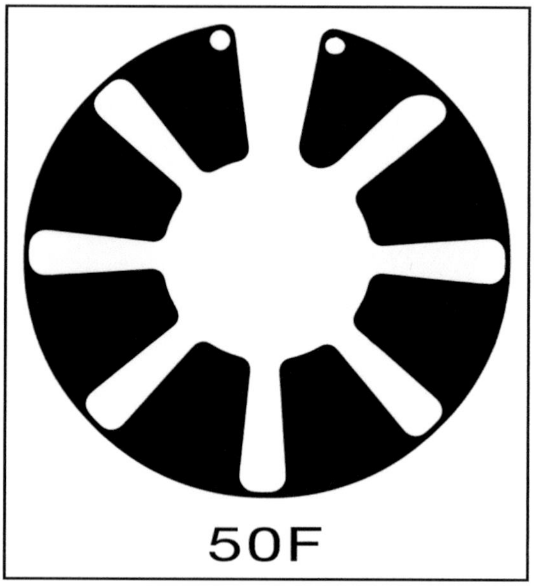

Figure 9-2. This 50F modified capsular tension ring (Morcher GmbH) contains multiple black occluder paddles. Two devices must be implanted inside the capsular bag and the occluder paddles on 1 ring must be aligned with the slit spaces on the other ring to create a fixed 4-mm pupil. (Reprinted with permission from Morcher GmbH.)

are 4 companies that manufacture devices for iris reconstruction. They include Morcher GmbH, Ophtec BV, HumanOptics AG, and Reper-NN Ltd. We have no experience with Reper as they are relatively new to the market. The devices fall broadly into 2 categories: modified capsular tension rings and artificial iris devices, which include iris reconstruction lenses.

Modified Capsular Tension Rings

In some cases, it is possible to keep light from entering an eye through an iris defect by placing a modified capsular tension ring inside the capsular bag and positioning an occluder paddle behind the iris defect (Figure 9-1). This approach requires an intact capsular bag and simultaneous cataract surgery.

An alternative approach to purse string pupilloplasty is capsular bag implantation of 2 modified capsular tension rings with multiple black occluder paddles (Figure 9-2). This approach also works

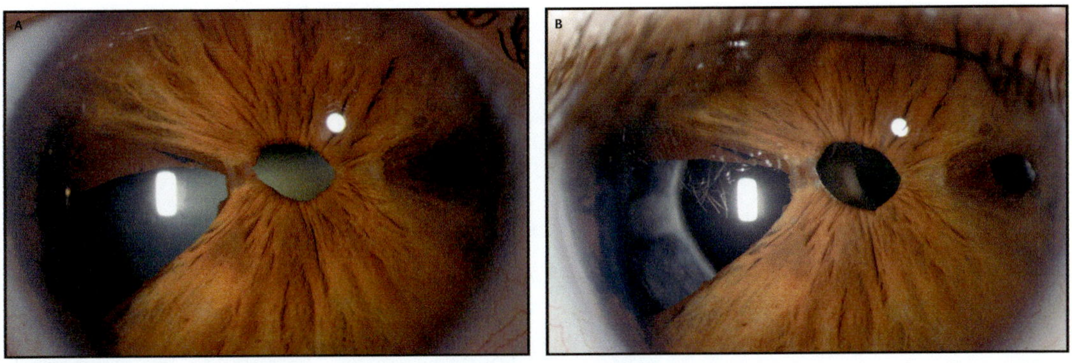

Figure 9-3. (A) This patient suffered from incomplete aniridia. He had full-thickness nasal and temporal iris defects. (B) At the time of cataract surgery, 2 Morcher 50F modified capsular tension rings were implanted inside the capsular bag, immediately anterior to the IOL. They kept him from experiencing postoperative photophobia or glare sensitivity by preventing incoming light from hitting the edge of the IOL.

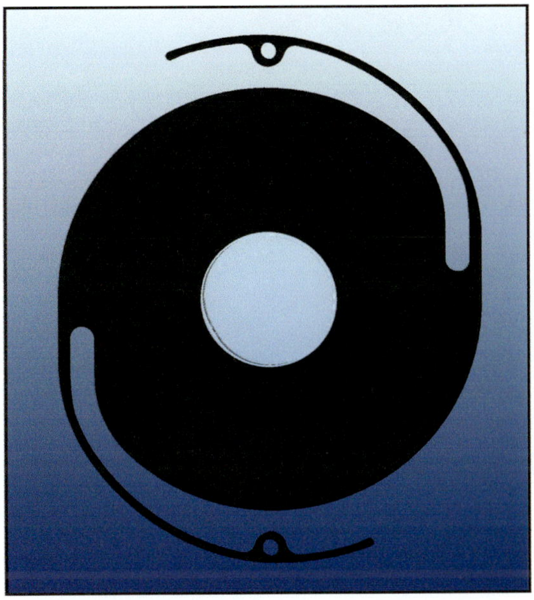

Figure 9-4. This 67B iris reconstruction lens (Morcher GmbH) contains a 3-mm optic, a 10-mm black iris diaphragm, and two 12.5-mm haptics with suture fixation eyelets. (Reprinted with permission from Morcher GmbH.)

if the iris has multiple mid-peripheral transillumination defects. It requires an intact capsular bag and simultaneous cataract surgery. The result is a fixed 4-mm pupil.

Figure 9-3 shows an eye with incomplete congenital aniridia and 2 iris defects that were managed by capsular bag implantation of 2 modified capsular tension rings containing multiple black occluder paddles.

Morcher Devices

Morcher GmbH manufactures a series of iris reconstruction lenses. These devices consist of a clear central optic surrounded by a black diaphragm and 2 haptics. Individual devices vary by the size of their optic and the diameter of their haptics. We have experience with the model 67B at our institution (Figure 9-4), although other models are available commercially. The model 67B has a 3-mm diameter optic, a 10-mm black iris diaphragm, and a haptic diameter of 12.5 mm. It is made for implantation within the ciliary sulcus, either passively, if there is capsular support, or by the use of scleral sutures. These devices can be placed into eyes affected by congenital or acquired aniridia

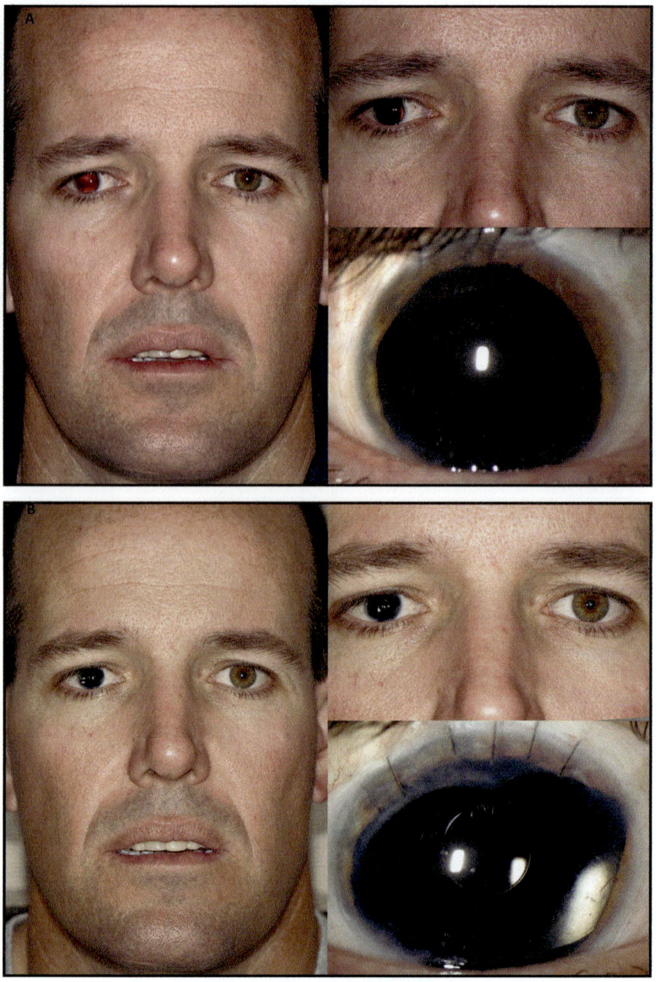

Figure 9-5. (A) This man suffered a bottle rocket injury to his right eye. In the injury, he experienced a corneal laceration, hyphema, vitreous hemorrhage, retinal tears, a traumatic cataract, and secondary glaucoma. Prior to presentation, he underwent a pars plana vitrectomy lensectomy, scleral buckling, retinal cryopexy, and air-fluid exchange, followed some time later by glaucoma seton implantation. (B) His aphakia and near-complete aniridia were treated by scleral suture fixation of a 67B iris reconstruction lens.

that is either partial or complete. If any posterior synechiae are present, they must be broken to ensure proper centration of the device.

Figure 9-5 shows before and after photos of a patient with a large iris defect who was surgically aphakic at the time of presentation.

Ophtec Devices

Ophtec BV manufactures aniridia implants for iris reconstruction and aphakia correction. The implants are 2-piece devices that are made from clear and colored ultraviolet light-absorbing polymethyl methacrylate. The irises are available in monochromatic brown, blue, or green colors. The artificial iris is 9.0 mm in diameter and the central optic is 4.0 mm in diameter. Available lens powers range from +10.0 to +30.0 diopters (D) in 0.5 D increments. The device has 2 C-loop haptics, each with an eyelet at the apex to provide the option for suture fixation to the sclera. These devices are designed for implantation into aphakic eyes, but they can also be used in piggyback manner. They can be suture-fixated to the sclera, placed passively in the sulcus, or implanted within the capsular bag.

Figure 9-6 shows before and after photos of a patient with a history of radial and astigmatic keratotomy in his left eye who experienced a subsequent fist injury, resulting in globe rupture.

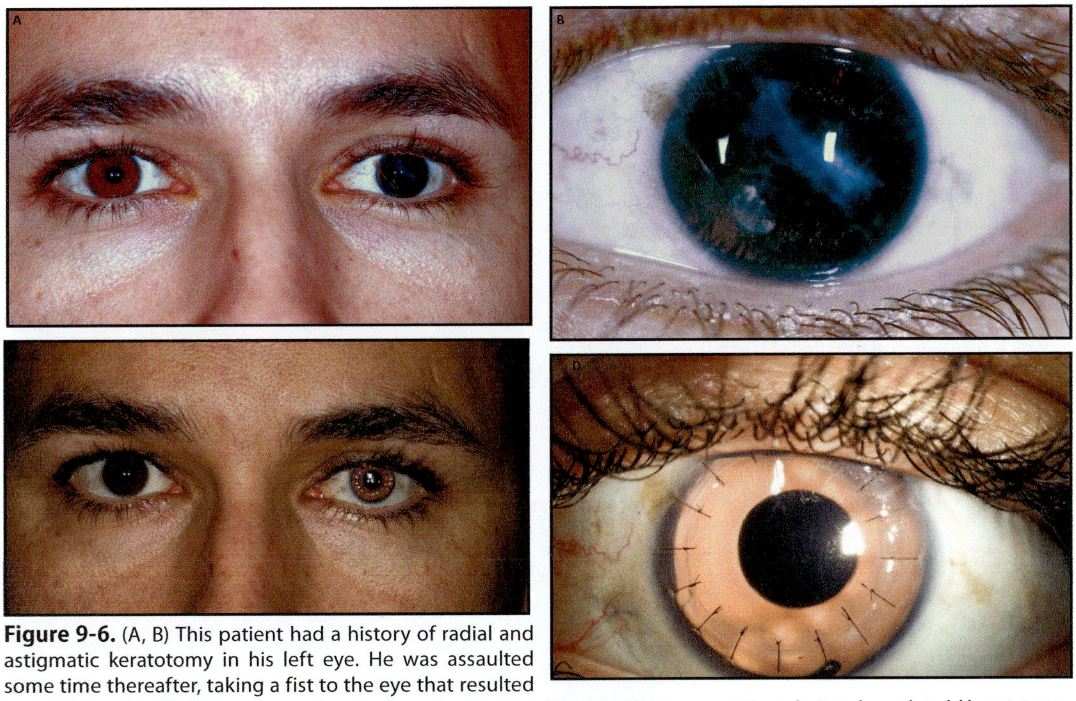

Figure 9-6. (A, B) This patient had a history of radial and astigmatic keratotomy in his left eye. He was assaulted some time thereafter, taking a fist to the eye that resulted in multiple orbital fractures, corneal rupture, and extrusion of the iris. The preoperative photos show the old keratotomy scars and a healed 6-mm central corneal laceration. He was completely aniridic. What was left of his crystalline lens was scarred to the posterior cornea at the time of presentation. (C, D) He underwent penetrating keratoplasty, anterior vitrectomy, and implantation with scleral suture fixation of a brown 311 iris reconstruction lens (Ophtec).

HumanOptics Device

HumanOptics AG is the distributor of a custom artificial iris device manufactured by Dr. Schmidt Intraokularinsen (Video 9-2). It is a foldable, custom-painted iris prosthesis made from silicone. The devices are individually hand-painted based on a patients' residual iris fellow eye photographs, when available. The implant is foldable and thus requires only a small incision for insertion. The device is intended for implantation in pseudophakic or aphakic eyes only. It can be trephined and placed in the capsular bag in front of an intraocular lens (IOL). It can also be fixated passively within the sulcus. In the absence of an intact capsular bag, it can be sutured to the sclera directly or it can be sutured to an IOL, which is then sutured to the sclera. The device has an overall diameter of 12.8 mm and a fixed pupil size of 3.35 mm.[18]

Figure 9-7 shows before and after photos of a patient with a large nasal iris defect that was repaired by HumanOptics artificial iris device implantation.

Conclusion

Iris repair or reconstruction is an advanced surgical procedure that can be undertaken with sutures or iris prostheses (see Video 9-1). While polypropylene suture repair is readily available, its usefulness is limited to the repair of small defects, iridodialyses, and atonic pupils. Artificial iris devices can correct larger defects, but they are currently restricted in the United States and some other markets. Surgical planning should consider not only the specific technique to be used but also concurrent ocular comorbidities. Successful repair can result in significant cosmetic and functional improvement.

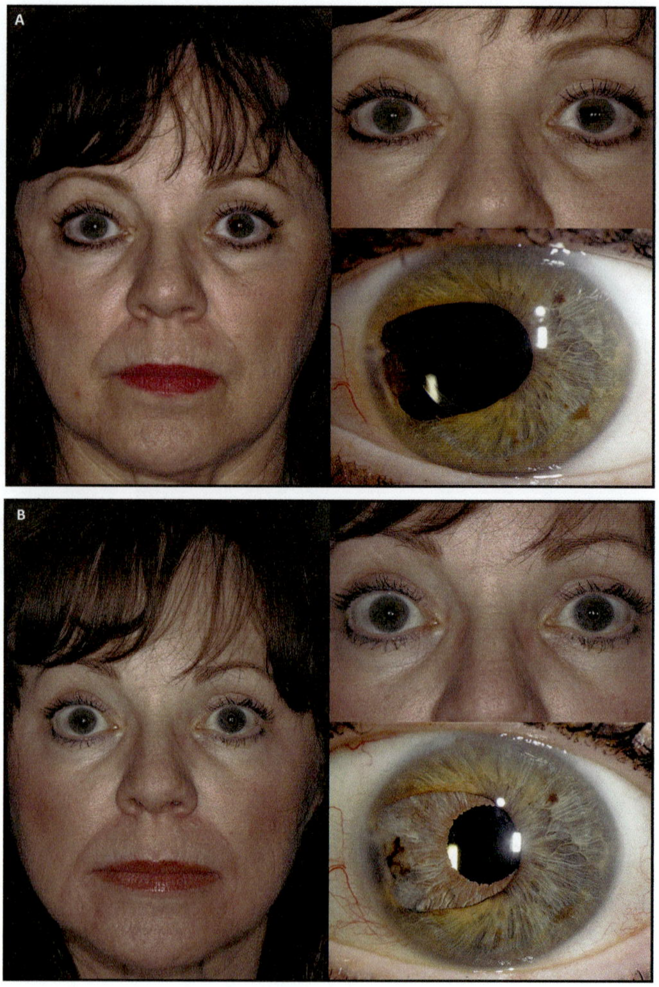

Figure 9-7. (A) This woman suffered a penetrating scissors injury to her left eye when she was 2.5 years old. She underwent eye muscle surgery a few years later. Prior to presentation at our office, she underwent cataract extraction with toric posterior chamber intraocular lens (PC IOL) implantation. Despite excellent uncorrected distance visual acuity, she suffered from intolerable nighttime glare sensitivity and could not drive at night. (B) A HumanOptics custom artificial iris device was placed passively into the ciliary sulcus, producing a very nice cosmetic and functional result.

Case Presentation 1

Aniridia Rings

Priya Narang, MS; Ashvin Agarwal, MBBS, MS; and Amar Agarwal, MS, FRCS, FRCOphth

A patient presented with subluxated cataract, traumatic mydriasis and iris defect in 1 quadrant. Capsulorrhexis was performed and a capsular tension ring was inserted into the capsular bag for stabilization. Following removal of cataract, 2 modified capsular tension rings with multiple black occluder paddles (Figure 9-8) were implanted into the capsular bag. This approach worked effectively to stabilize the capsular bag as well as prevent glare and photophobia (Video 9-3).

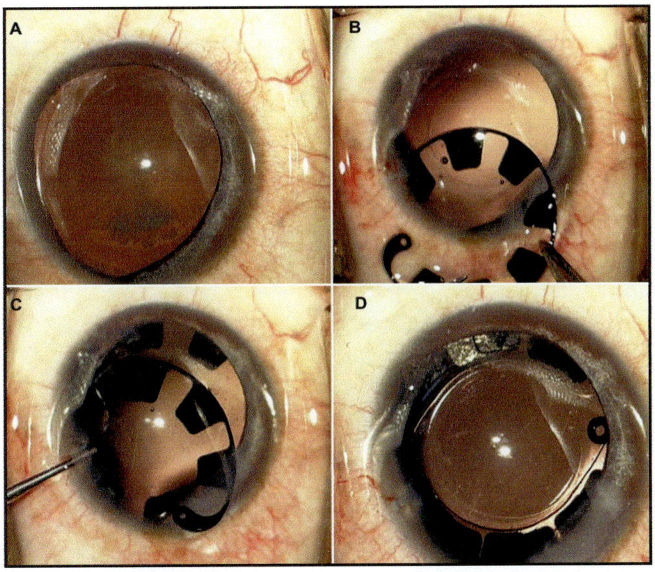

Figure 9-8. Implantation of modified capsular tension ring with occluders for iris defect. (A) A case with subluxated cataract and iris defect with traumatic mydriasis. (B) The first modified capsular tension ring with occluder being implanted into the capsular bag. (C) The second occluder ring being placed into the capsular bag. (D) Both occluder rings are placed in the capsular bag in a way that the occluder paddles do not overlap but lie adjacent to each other. This ensures blockage of light rays from the peripheral area of iris defect.

Case Presentation 2

Sutured Artificial Iris

Michael E. Snyder, MD

A patient presented with poor vision and photic symptoms due to traumatic aniridia and traumatic aphakia with a small opening in the posterior capsule. There was a well healed, full-thickness sectoral peripheral corneal scar. The patient elected to have a 3-piece foldable IOL placed along with custom-made iris prosthesis (CustomFlex ArtificialIris, HumanOptics AG) into the sulcus. This artificial iris was cut using a trephine according to the size required for the particular eye. It was then sutured to the sclera using expanded polytetrafluoroethylene suture (Gore-Tex) after injecting it inside the anterior chamber through an injector (Figure 9-9 and Video 9-4).

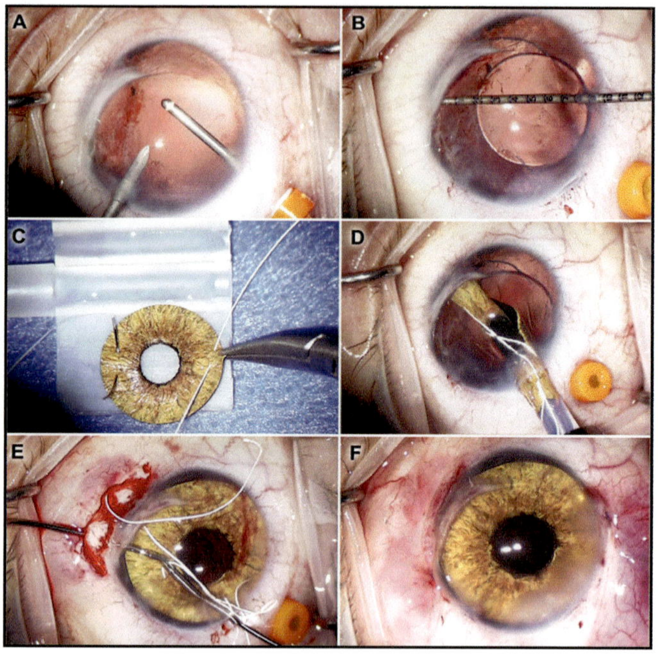

Figure 9-9. Sutured artificial iris. (A) Traumatic aniridia with aphakia. (B) Three-piece PC IOL implanted in sulcus with optic capture through a vitrector-fashioned posterior capsulorrhexis and measurement taken for correct size trephination required of the artificial iris. (C) Artificial iris, already cut to size with trephine and sutured with 2 horizontal mattress Gore-Tex sutures placed through the periphery of the device. (D) Artificial iris (with pre-placed sutures) injected into the anterior chamber through an injector. (E) Artificial iris device is unfolded and the sutures retrieved through the sclera. (F) Artificial iris fixated and aphakia solved at the same time.

Case Presentation 3

Artificial Iris With Yamane Technique. Double-Needle Scleral Intraocular Lens and Artificial Iris Fixation

Vladimir Pfeifer, MD, FEBOS-CR

A patient presented with aniridia and aphakia. This patient needed an artificial iris with a secondary IOL. There was no capsule present. A 3-piece IOL was passed through an artificial iris. Subsequently, the entire artificial iris/IOL complex was passed into the anterior chamber. The Yamane technique was performed to stabilize it (Figure 9-10 and Video 9-5).

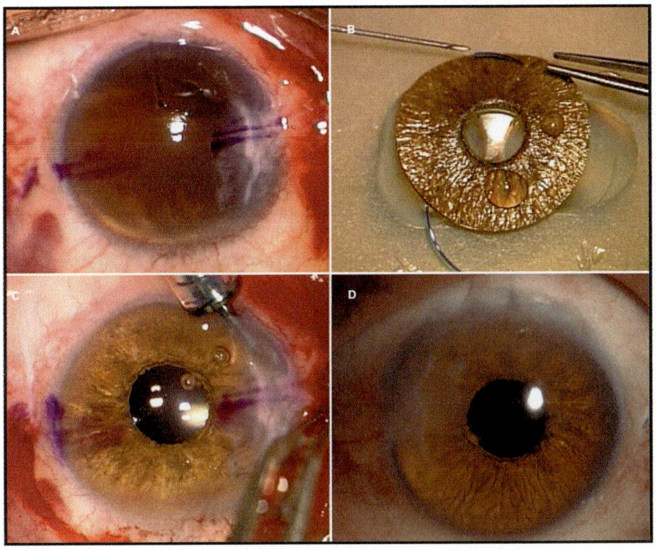

Figure 9-10. Artificial iris with Yamane technique. Double-needle scleral IOL and artificial iris fixation. (A) Traumatic aniridia with aphakia. (B) A 3-piece PC IOL locked and passed through the artificial iris. (C) Artificial iris cut with trephine and the 3-piece IOL passed into the anterior chamber. Yamane technique performed. (D) Postoperative photo shows aniridia solved with a secondary IOL implanted.

References

1. Burk SE, Da Mata AP, Snyder ME, Cionni RJ, Cohen JS, Osher RH. Prosthetic iris implantation for congenital, traumatic, or functional iris deficiencies. *J Cataract Refract Surg.* 2001;27:1732-1740.
2. Karatza EC, Burk SE, Snyder ME, Osher RH. Outcomes of prosthetic iris implantation in patients with albinism. *J Cataract Refract Surg.* 2007;33:1763-1769.
3. Date RC, Olson MD, Shah M, Masket S, Miller KM. Outcomes of a modified capsular tension ring with a single black occluder paddle for eyes with congenital and acquired iris defects: report 2. *J Cataract Refract Surg.* 2015;41:1934-1944.
4. Miller KM, Nicoli CM, Olson MD, Shah M, Masket S. Outcomes of implantation of modified capsule tension rings with multiple black occluder paddles for eyes with congenital and acquired iris defects: report 3. *J Cataract Refract Surg.* 2016;42:870-878.
5. McCannel MA. A retrievable suture idea for anterior uveal problems. *Ophthalmic Surg.* 1976; 7:98-103.
6. Siepser SB. The closed chamber slipping suture technique for iris repair. *Ann Ophthalmol.* 1994;26:71-72.
7. Osher RH, Snyder ME, Cionni RJ. Modification of the Siepser slip-knot technique. *J Cataract Refract Surg.* 2005;31:1098-1100.
8. Kaufman SC, Insler MS. Surgical repair of a traumatic iridodialysis. *Ophthalmic Surg Lasers.* 1996;27:963-966.
9. Hoffman RS, Fine IH, Packer M. Scleral fixation without conjunctival dissection. *J Cataract Refract Surg.* 2006;32:1907-1912.
10. Snyder ME, Lindsell LB. Nonappositional repair of iridodialysis. *J Cataract Refract Surg.* 2011;37:625-628.
11. Brown SM. A technique for repair of iridodialysis in children. *JAAPOS.* 1998;2:380-382.
12. Ogawa GS. The iris cerclage suture for permanent mydriasis: a running suture technique. *Ophthalmic Surg Lasers.* 1998;29:1001-1009.
13. Mansour AM, Ahmed II, Eadie B, et al. Iritis, glaucoma and corneal decompensation associated with BrightOcular cosmetic iris implant. *Br J Ophthalmol.* 2016;100:1098-1101.
14. Hoguet A, Ritterband D, Koplin R, Wu E, Raviv T, Aljian J, Seedor J. Serious ocular complications of cosmetic iris implants in 14 eyes. *J Cataract Refract Surg.* 2012;38:387-393.
15. Olson MD, Masket S, Miller KM. Interim results of a compassionate-use clinical trial of Morcher iris diaphragm implantation: report 1. *J Cataract Refract Surg.* 2008;34:1674-1680.
16. Aslam SA, Wong SC, Ficker LA, MacLaren RE. Implantation of the black diaphragm intraocular lens in congenital and traumatic aniridia. *Ophthalmology.* 2008;115:1705-1712.
17. Price MO, Price FW Jr, Chang DF, Kelley K, Olson MD, Miller KM. Ophtec iris reconstruction lens United States clinical trial phase I. *Ophthalmology.* 2004;111:1847-1852.
18. Mayer CS, Reznicek L, Hoffmann AE. Pupillary reconstruction and outcome after artificial iris implantation. *Ophthalmology.* 2016123:1011-1018.

Please visit www.routledge.com/9781630917265

to access additional material.

10

Twofold Technique for Iridodialysis Repair

Priya Narang, MS; Ashvin Agarwal, MBBS, MS; and Amar Agarwal, MS, FRCS, FRCOphth

Keywords

hang-back technique, iridodialysis, iris repair, non-appositional repair, single-pass four-throw pupilloplasty, twofold technique

Iridodialysis

The term *iridodialysis* refers to the disinsertion of the iris root from its base. It is mostly traumatic in nature (Figure 10-1), but can also be iatrogenic. It is rarely congenital in origin. It is imperative to repair an iridodialysis as it can lead to monocular diplopia, glare, or photophobia. The presence or absence of symptoms depends upon the amount of iridodialysis and its relevant position. For a small defect with less than 1 clock hour, superior iridodialysis can be left in situ as it does not produce any symptoms because the upper eyelid covers up the superior defect. However, if it is present in other quadrants and is more than 1 clock hour, iris base repair should be performed.

Twofold Technique

Various techniques have been described in peer-reviewed literature for the repair of iridodialysis.[1-8] The twofold technique[9] combines the non-appositional[6] technique with the single-pass four-throw (SFT) pupilloplasty[10] technique that works effectively in iridodialysis cases with varied degrees of severity.

Agarwal A, Agarwal A, eds. *Mastering Iris Repair: A Video Textbook of Iris Repair and Pupilloplasty Techniques* (pp 97-116).

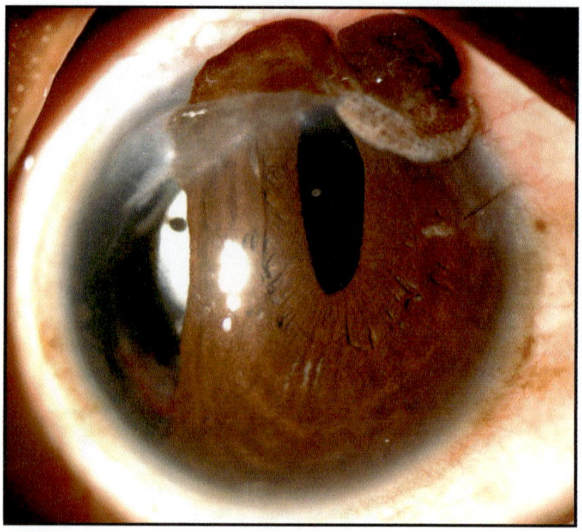

Figure 10-1. Iridodialysis with iris prolapse due to injury.

Clinically, depending upon the amount of iris disinsertion and the variation in the application of the twofold technique, we have classified iridodialysis into the following 3 types:

1. Massive (> 120 degrees)
2. Moderate (45 to 120 degrees)
3. Minimal (< 45 degrees)

Massive Iridodialysis

In cases with massive iridodialysis, the peripheral iris is reapposed to the scleral base with the non-appositional technique (hang-back technique) as described by Snyder and Lindsell.[6] A 10-0 polypropylene double-armed suture attached to a long-armed needle is passed (Figure 10-2) after engaging the peripheral iris into the corresponding scleral base area (see Figures 10-2 through 10-6). The second arm of the needle is then passed through the adjacent peripheral iris tissue. Both the suture ends are pulled and tied, and the knot is buried into the scleral groove. In some cases with massive iridodialysis, the iris tissue is absent or is too minimal to be reapposed. In such cases, SFT is performed (see Figure 10-3) to cover up the areas of iris defect. With the combined approach, the iris and pupil can be made to appear nearly normal (see Figure 10-5 and Video 10-1).

Moderate Iridodialysis

In cases with moderate iridodialysis (Figures 10-7 through 10-10), the hang-back technique (Figures 10-11 through 10-14) can be performed followed by a glued intraocular lens (IOL) implantation if eye is aphakic. SFT pupilloplasty is then performed (Figures 10-15 through 10-17). Alternatively, depending on the case, SFT can be performed initially along the base of disinserted iris tissue. The 10-0 suture needle is passed in a way that approximates the adjacent and corresponding iris tissue. The advantage in doing so is that the gap of iris defect is decreased. Non-appositional repair can then be performed to reaffix the iris tissue to its base (Figure 10-18).

Minimal Iridodialysis

In cases with minimal iridodialysis, non-appositional repair is performed followed by SFT if corectopia is noticed (Figures 10-19 and 10-20). This can be understood via the illustrations in Figures 10-21 through 10-23.

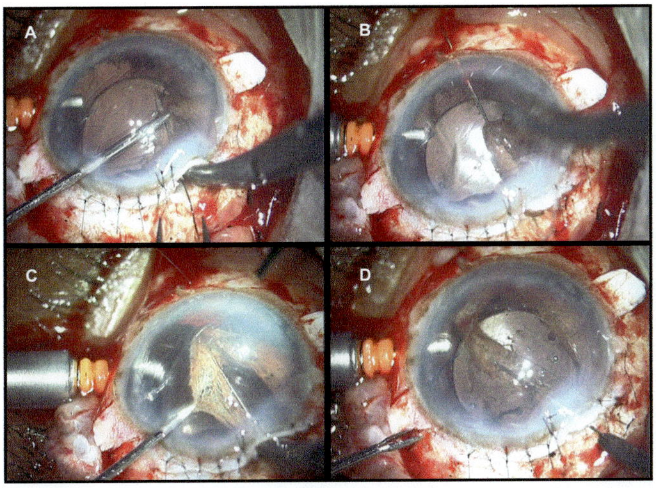

Figure 10-2. Twofold technique for traumatic massive iridodialysis (A) The iris tissue is repositioned inside the anterior chamber and the 10-0 double-armed suture attached to the long straight needle is passed through the base of the disinserted iris tissue. (B) The 10-0 needle is passed through the scleral wall at a distance of around 1.5 mm from the limbus. (C) The second arm of the suture is passed through the iris tissue adjacent to the previous pass. The edge of iris tissue is held with an end-opening forceps to facilitate the passage of 10-0 needle. The knot is then tied and the iris tissue is apposed to the scleral wall. (D) Another double-armed 10-0 suture attached to the long needle is passed through the adjacent iris tissue and non-appositional repair is performed. (Republished with permission of Elsevier, from Narang P, Agarwal A, Agarwal A, Agarwal A. Twofold technique of nonappositional repair with single-pass four-throw pupilloplasty for iridodialysis. *J Cataract Refract Surg*, 44[12];2018; permission conveyed through Copyright Clearance Center, Inc.)

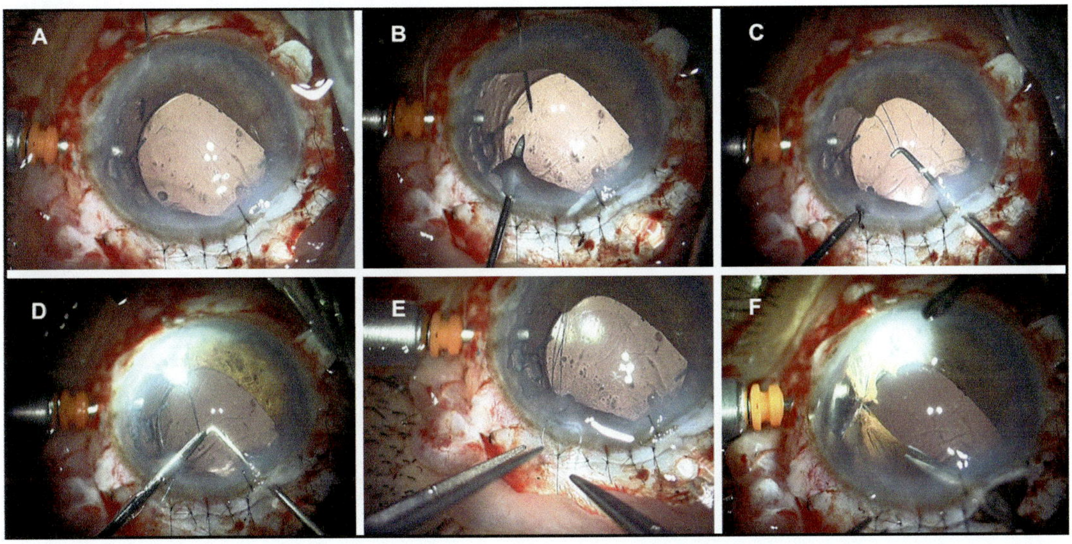

Figure 10-3. Twofold technique for traumatic massive iridodialysis. (A) Paracentesis incision is created and SFT pupilloplasty procedure begins with a 10-0 single-armed suture attached to the long needle passed through the proximal iris tissue. (B) A 26-gauge needle is introduced from the paracentesis incision from the opposite side that is passed through the distal iris tissue. (C) The 10-0 needle is threaded into the barrel of the 26-gauge needle, and it is then withdrawn. A Sinskey hook is passed and a loop of the suture is withdrawn in to the anterior chamber. (D) The loop is held with an end-opening forceps and is withdrawn outside the anterior chamber. (E) The suture end is passed through the loop and 4 throws are taken. (F) Both the suture ends are pulled and the iris tissue is approximated. The suture ends are cut with microscissors. (Republished with permission of Elsevier, from Narang P, Agarwal A, Agarwal A, Agarwal A. Twofold technique of nonappositional repair with single-pass four-throw pupilloplasty for iridodialysis. *J Cataract Refract Surg*, 44[12];2018; permission conveyed through Copyright Clearance Center, Inc.)

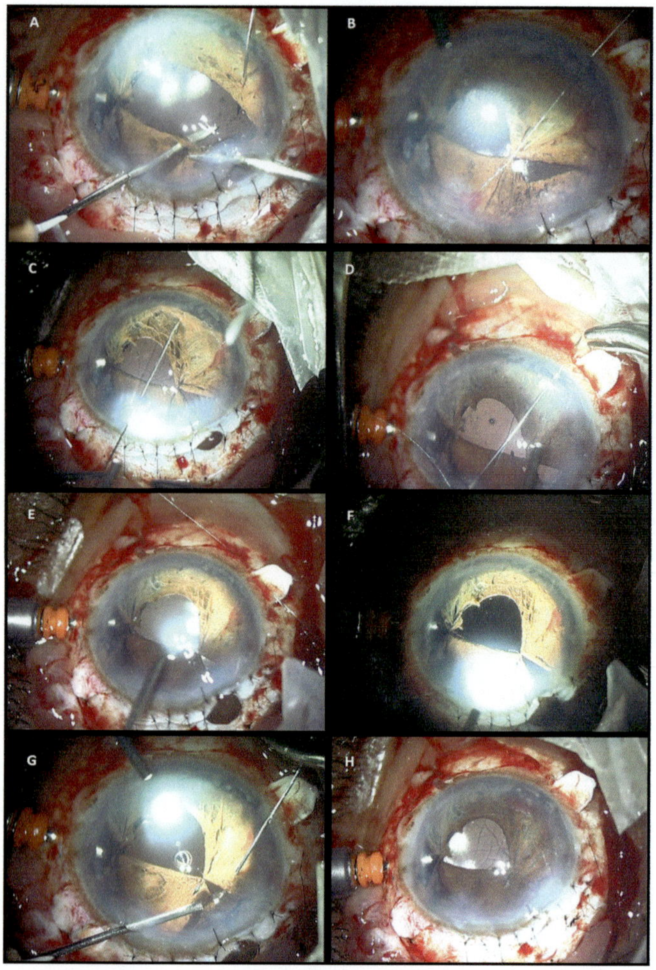

Figure 10-4. Twofold technique for traumatic massive iridodialysis. (A) SFT is performed in the opposite quadrant. (B) Iris tissue is apposed and central pupillary contour is achieved. (C) Non-appositional repair is being performed in the remaining area of iridodialysis. (D) The second arm of 10-0 suture is passed through the adjacent iris tissue. (E) The knot is tied and buried in the scleral groove. (F) Effective functional pupil contour is achieved. (G) SFT pupilloplasty is performed to close the peripheral iris tissue gap. (H) Complete iris repair is achieved. (Republished with permission of Elsevier, from Narang P, Agarwal A, Agarwal A, Agarwal A. Twofold technique of nonappositional repair with single-pass four-throw pupilloplasty for iridodialysis. *J Cataract Refract Surg*, 44[12];2018; permission conveyed through Copyright Clearance Center, Inc.)

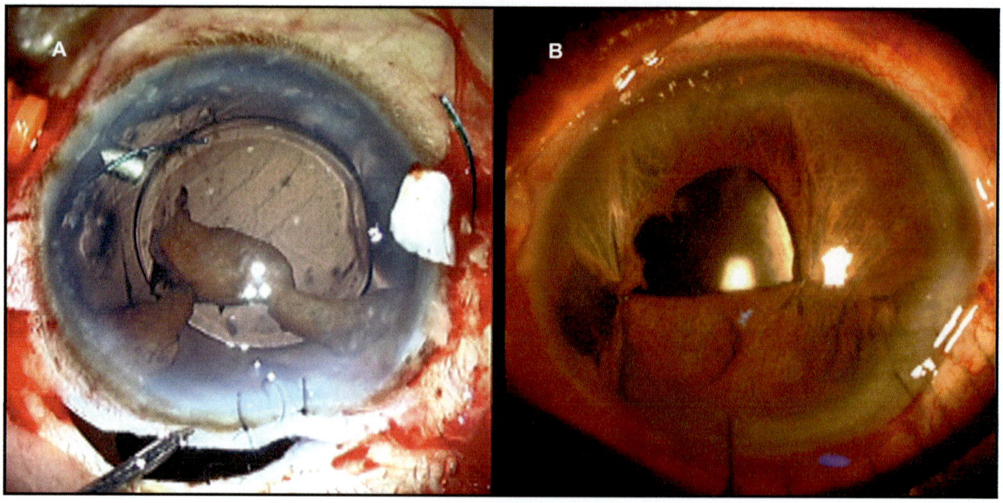

Figure 10-5. (A) Preoperative image of a case with massive iridodialysis. (B) Postoperative image of the case following twofold technique. (Republished with permission of Elsevier, from Narang P, Agarwal A, Agarwal A, Agarwal A. Twofold technique of nonappositional repair with single-pass four-throw pupilloplasty for iridodialysis. *J Cataract Refract Surg*, 44[12];2018; permission conveyed through Copyright Clearance Center, Inc.)

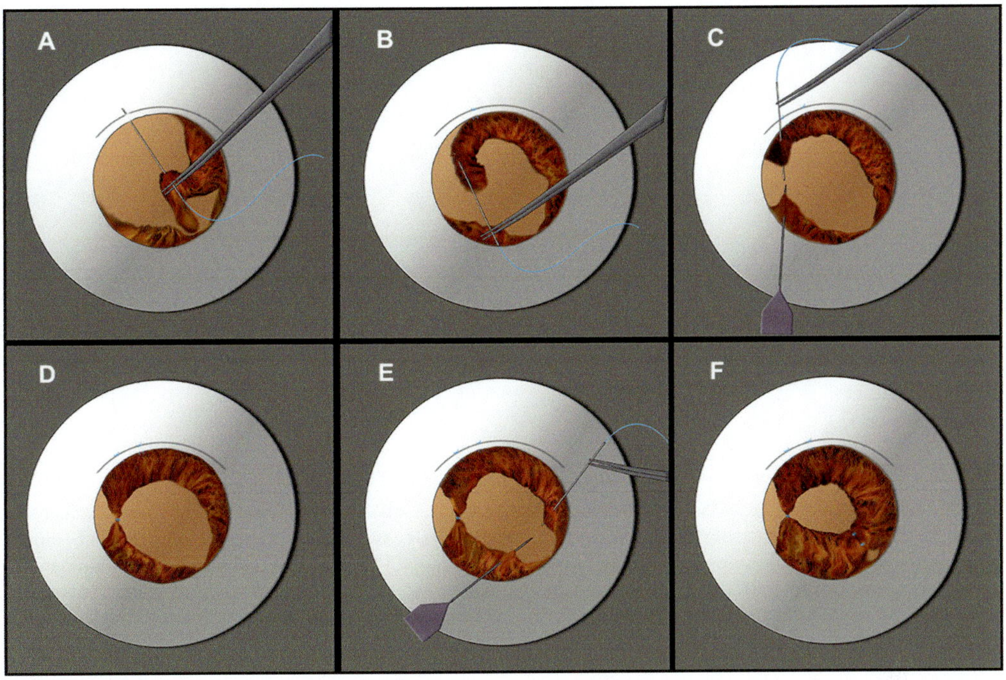

Figure 10-6. Illustration of twofold technique for massive iridodialysis. (A) Long-armed needle is passed through the edge of the peripheral iris tear tissue and the needle is exteriorized through the corresponding scleral area. (B) The adjacent iris tissue is also fixed to the scleral wall with the non-appositional technique. (C) Sectorial iris tissue defect is observed. SFT is performed by engaging the adjoining iris tissue. (D) The gap is closed or minimized with the SFT procedure, and pupil contour is achieved is one quadrant. (E) SFT is performed in the other quadrant. (F) Functional iris configuration is achieved in a case of massive iridodialysis. (Republished with permission of Elsevier, from Narang P, Agarwal A, Agarwal A, Agarwal A. Twofold technique of nonappositional repair with single-pass four-throw pupilloplasty for iridodialysis. *J Cataract Refract Surg,* 44[12];2018; permission conveyed through Copyright Clearance Center, Inc.)

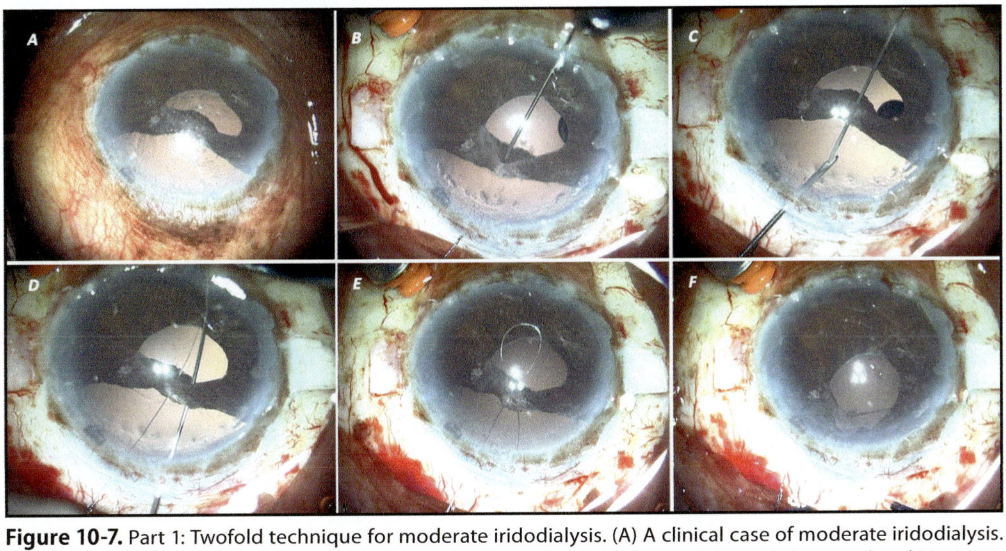

Figure 10-7. Part 1: Twofold technique for moderate iridodialysis. (A) A clinical case of moderate iridodialysis. (B) The 10-0 polypropylene suture attached to a long-armed needle is passed through the peripheral iris tissue. (C) A 26-gauge needle is introduced from the opposite side and the 10-0 needle is threaded into it. (D) The second arm of the needle is passed through the adjacent iris tissue. (E) Both the suture ends are pulled. This retracts the iris to its base. (F) The suture ends are tied and the knot is buried in the scleral groove.

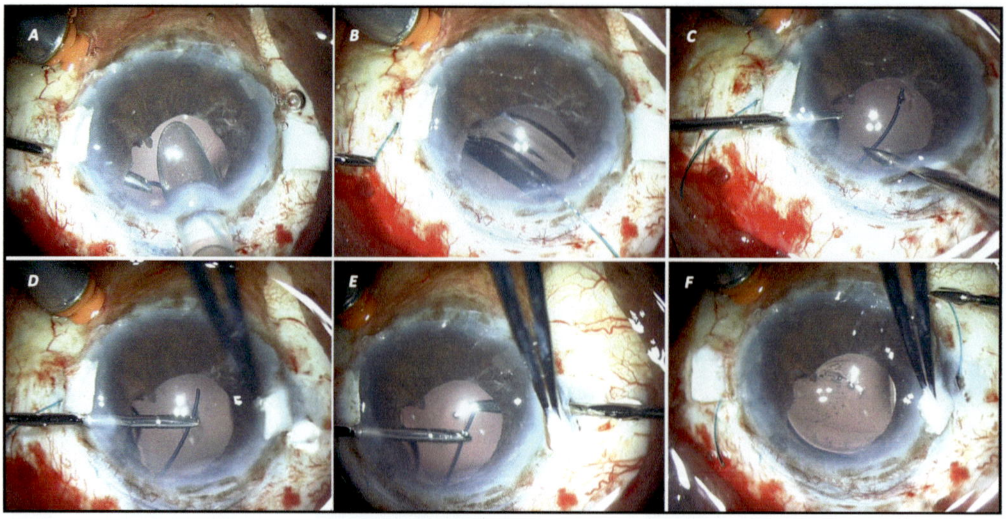

Figure 10-8. Part 2: Glued IOL performed in moderate iridodialysis case. (A) Glued IOL being implanted. Haptic caught with the glued IOL forceps. (B) Leading haptic externalized. (C) No assistant technique for trailing haptic. (D) Trailing haptic caught with the glued IOL forceps. (E) Handshake technique performed to grasp the trailing haptic. (F) Both haptics externalized. Subsequently, they are tucked in Scharioth pockets created by a 26-gauge needle and finally glued in using fibrin glue (Tisseel, Baxter).

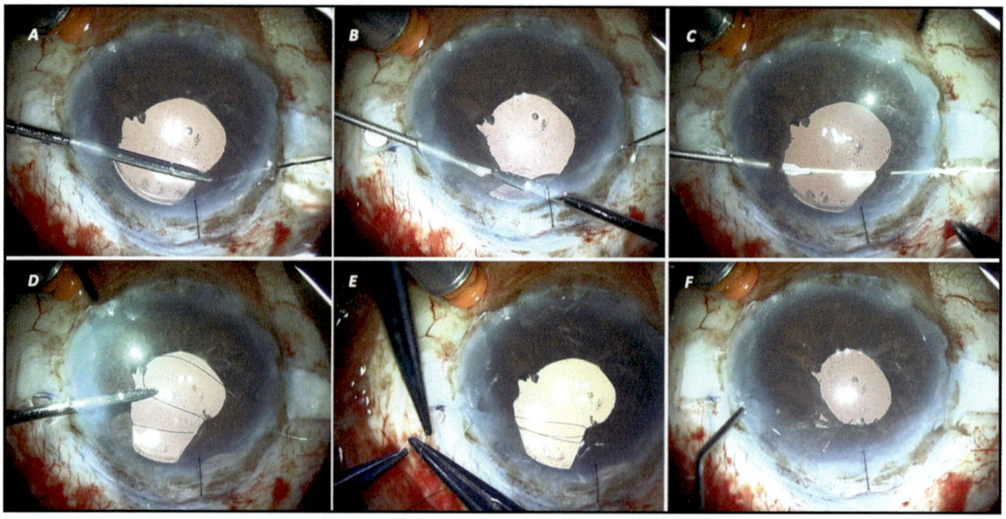

Figure 10-9. Part 3: Twofold technique for moderate iridodialysis. (A) To correct the updrawn pupil, a 10-0 Prolene (Ethicon) suture attached to the needle is passed through the proximal iris tissue. (B) A 26/30-gauge needle is passed from the paracentesis incision from the opposite side in a way that it engages the distal iris tissue to be approximated. (C) The 10-0 needle is threaded into the barrel of the 26-gauge needle, and the needle is pulled out of the anterior chamber. (D) The loop of the suture is withdrawn from the anterior chamber. (E) The suture end is passed from the loop 4 times. (F) Both the suture ends are pulled. This leads to sliding of the loop internally that approximates the concerned iris tissue.

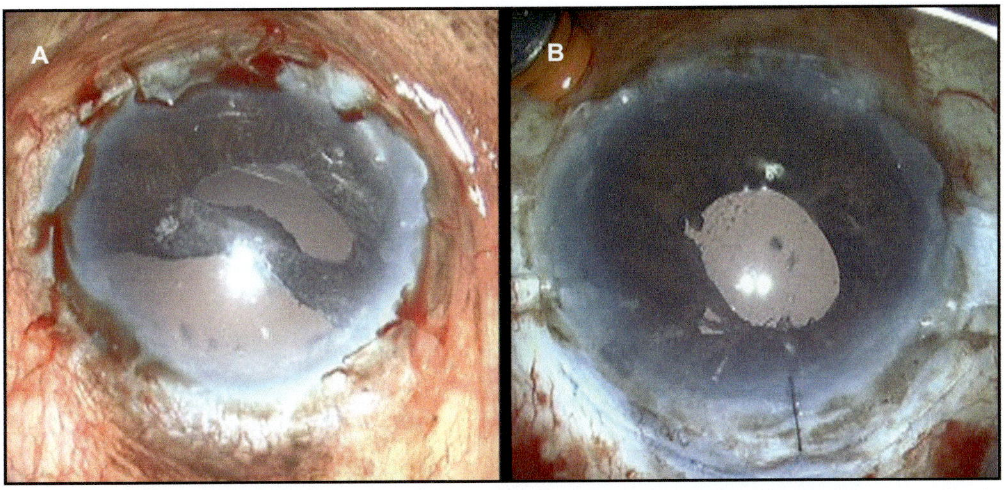

Figure 10-10. Part 4: Twofold technique for moderate iridodialysis. (A) Preoperative. (B) Immediately postoperative following twofold technique and glued IOL surgery.

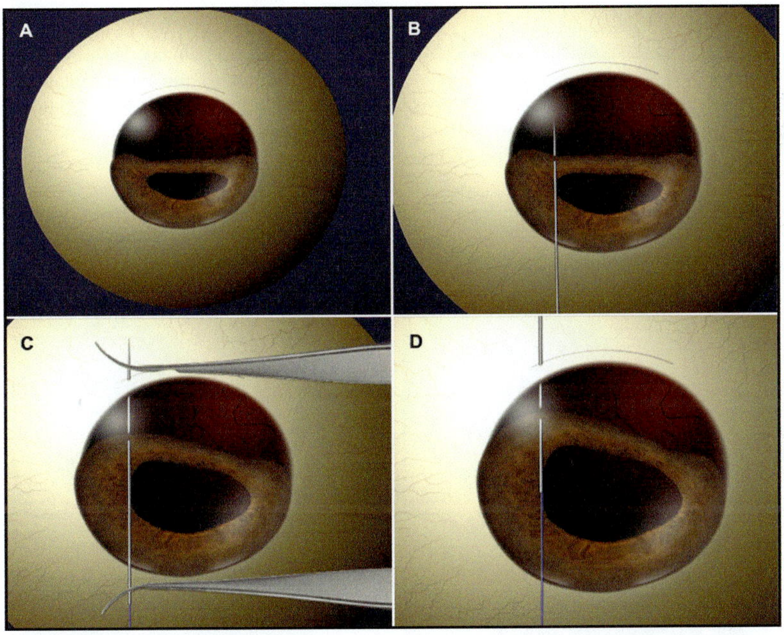

Figure 10-11. Part 1: Illustration showing the hang-back technique for iridodialysis. (A) Illustration showing iridodialysis. (B) The double-armed 10-0 polypropylene suture attached to the long-armed needle is passed through the peripheral iris tissue via a paracentesis. (C) The needle is brought out through a scleral groove. (D) The suture is brought out through the sclera.

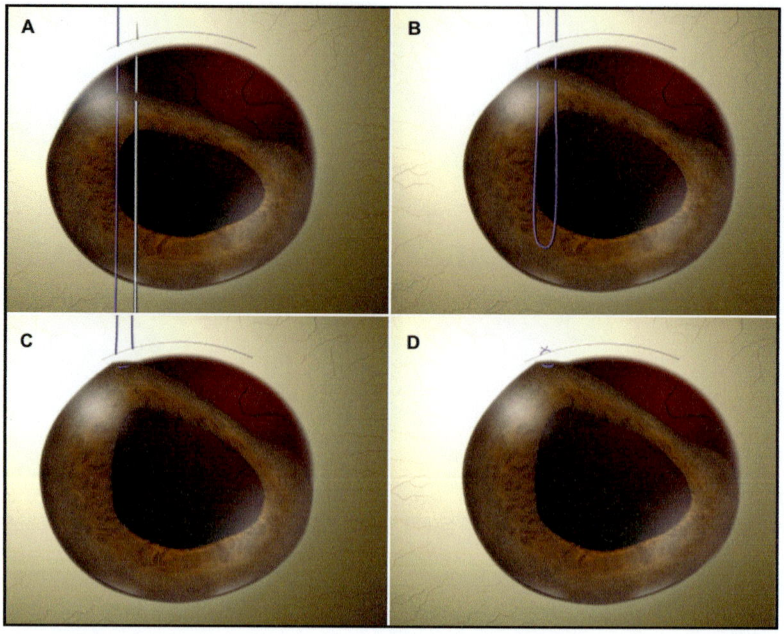

Figure 10-12. Part 2: Illustration showing the hang-back technique for iridodialysis. (A) The second arm of the needle is passed through the adjacent iris tissue. (B) Both the suture ends are pulled, which retracts the iris to the sclera. (C) The suture ends are pulled up. (D) The sutures are tied and the knot is buried in the scleral groove.

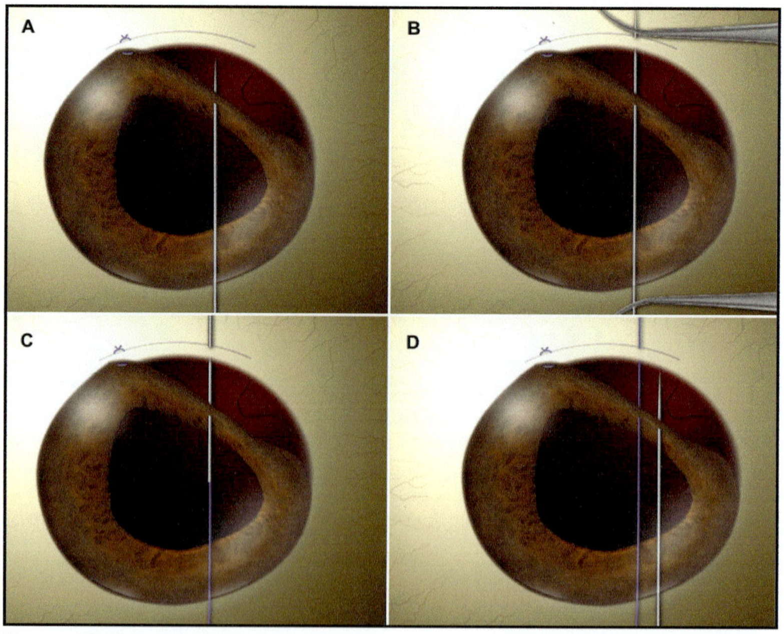

Figure 10-13. Part 3: Illustration showing the hang-back technique for iridodialysis. (A) The double-armed 10-0 polypropylene suture attached to the long-armed needle is passed through the peripheral iris tissue through a paracentesis in another area of the iridodialysis. (B) The needle is brought out through a scleral groove. (C) The suture is brought out through the sclera. (D) The other part of the double-armed needle is now passed through the peripheral iris.

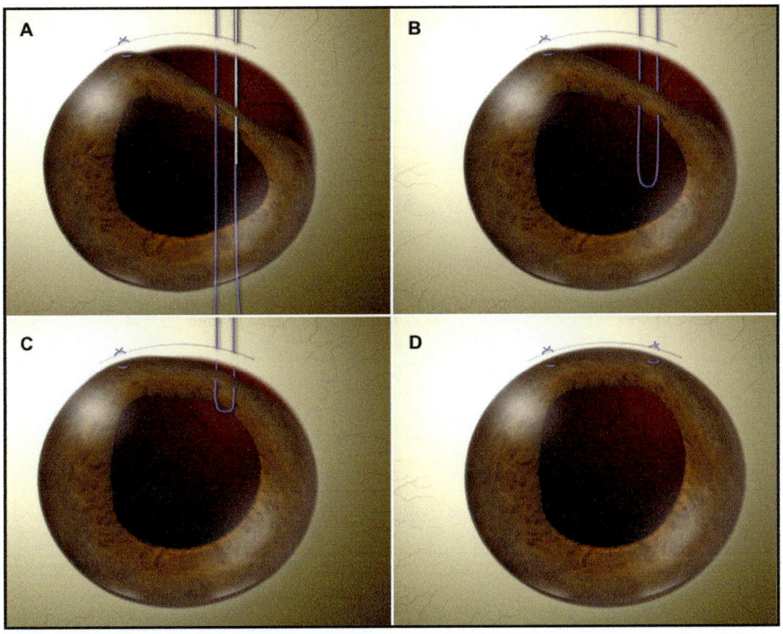

Figure 10-14. Part 4: Illustration showing the hang-back technique for iridodialysis. (A) Both suture ends are pulled, which retracts the iris. (B) Iris getting retracted. (C) Apposition of the iris to the sclera. (D) Suture tied.

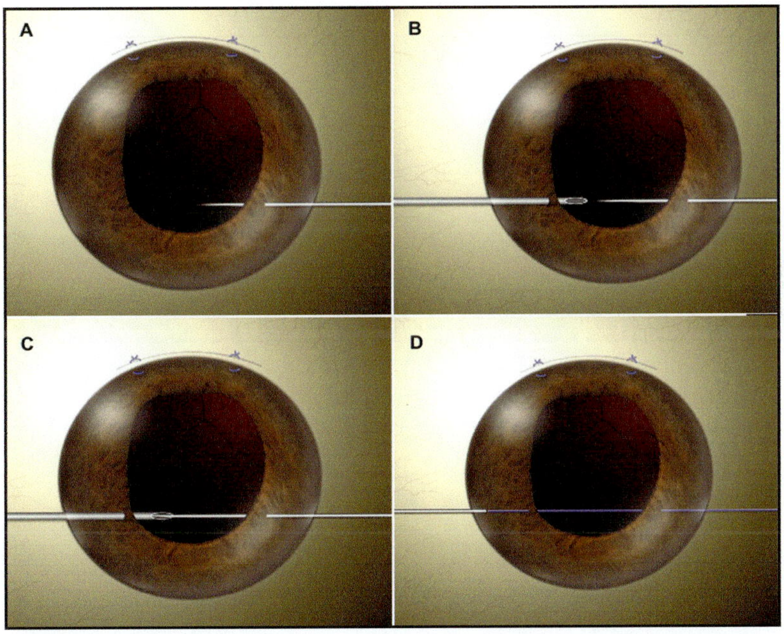

Figure 10-15. Part 1: Illustration showing the SFT pupilloplasty technique. (A) To correct the updrawn pupil, a 10-0 Prolene suture attached to the needle is passed through the proximal iris tissue. (B) A 26/30-gauge needle is passed from the paracentesis incision from the opposite side in a way that it engages the distal iris tissue to be approximated. (C) The 10-0 needle is threaded into the barrel of the 26-gauge needle and the needle is pulled out of the anterior chamber. (D) Suture being pulled out through the paracentesis.

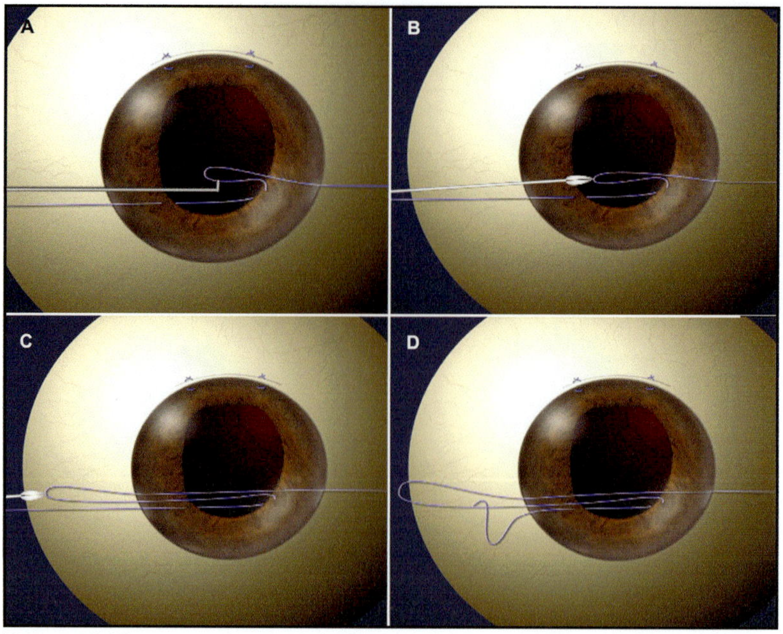

Figure 10-16. Part 2: Illustration showing the SFT pupilloplasty technique. (A) The loop of the suture is created using a dialer. (B) The loop of the suture is pulled on using the glued IOL forceps. (C) The loop of the suture is withdrawn from the anterior chamber. (D) Four throws are started on the loop that is outside.

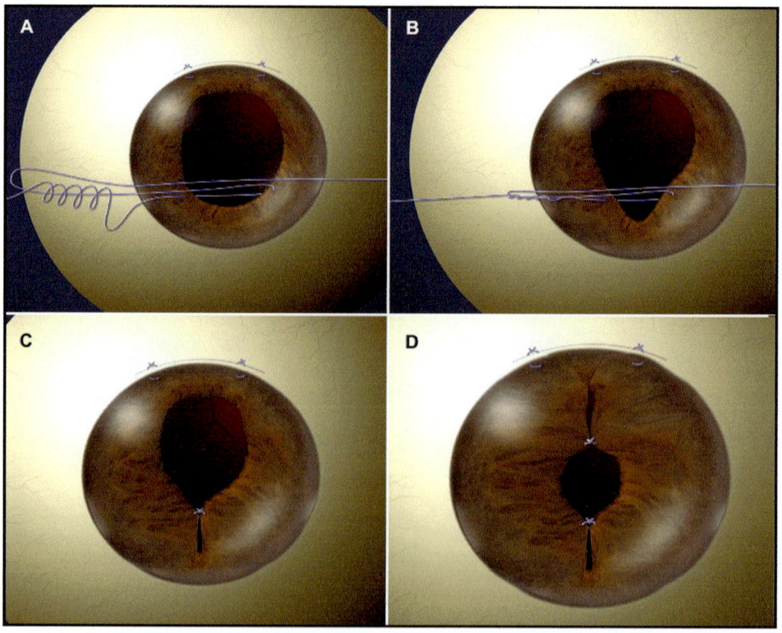

Figure 10-17. Part 3: Illustration showing the SFT pupilloplasty technique. (A) The suture end is passed from the loop 4 times. (B) The knot is slid into the eye by pulling at both ends. (C) SFT is completed and the ends of the suture cut with microscissors. (D) Same SFT procedure is performed at the other end to get a well-shaped pupil.

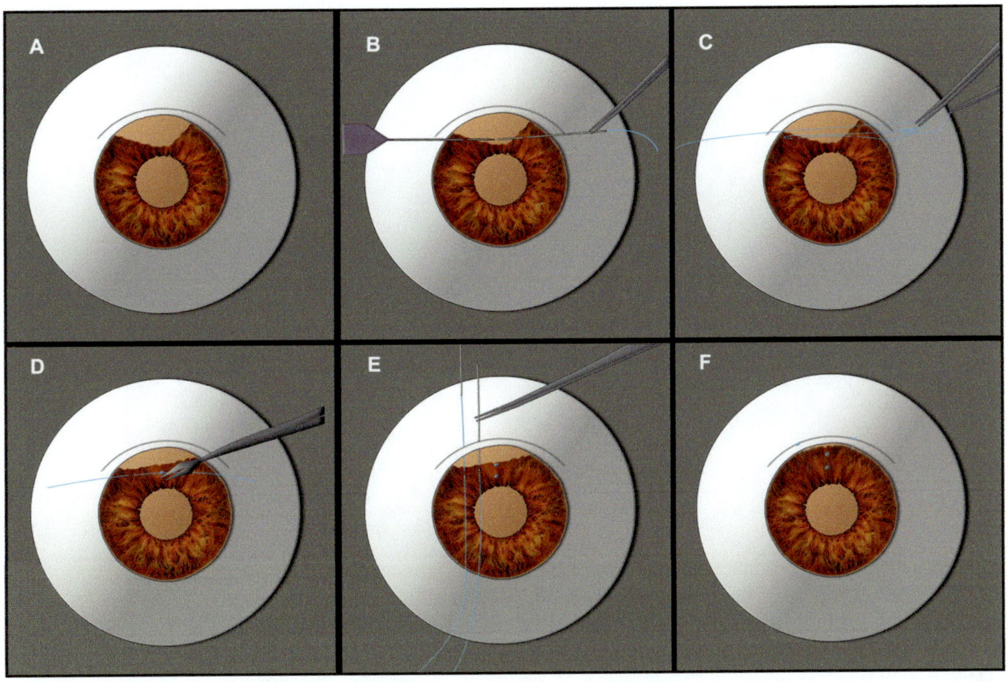

Figure 10-18. Illustration of twofold technique for moderate iridodialysis. (A) The image shows a moderate amount of iridodialysis. (B) A SFT procedure is being performed along the edge of the base of the iris tissue. A 10-0 suture on long-armed needle is passed from one side and a 26-gauge needle is passed from the corresponding iris tissue on the other side. (C) The 10-0 needle is threaded into the 26-gauge needle and is withdrawn from the anterior chamber. A loop of the suture is withdrawn from the anterior chamber and the suture end is passed from the loop taking 4 throws. (D) Both the suture ends are pulled and the iris tissue is approximated. The suture ends are cut with microscissors. Note the narrowing of the iridodialysis defect. (E) A 10-0 double-armed suture on a long needle is passed to reappose the peripheral iris defect with the hang-back technique. (F) The peripheral iris defect is sealed. (Republished with permission of Elsevier, from Narang P, Agarwal A, Agarwal A, Agarwal A. Twofold technique of nonappositional repair with single-pass four-throw pupilloplasty for iridodialysis. *J Cataract Refract Surg*, 44[12];2018; permission conveyed through Copyright Clearance Center, Inc.)

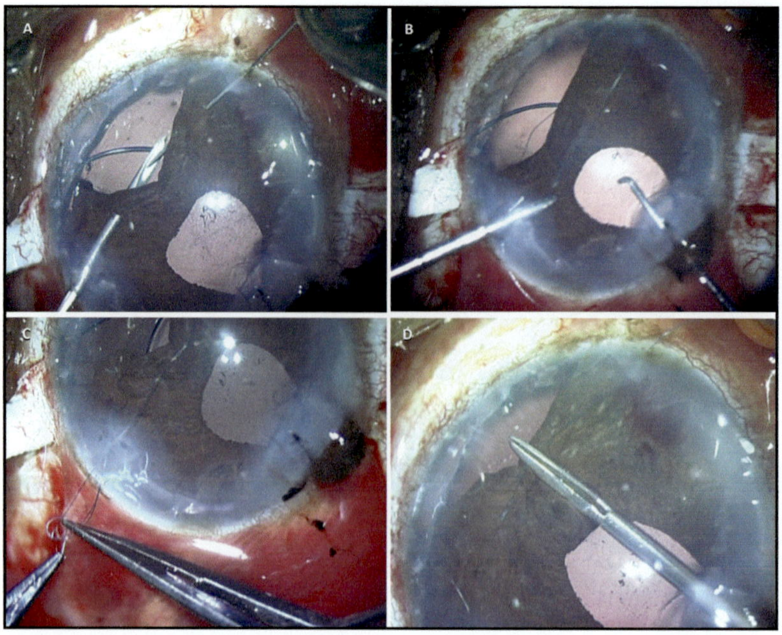

Figure 10-19. Part 1: Twofold technique for moderate to minimal iridodialysis. (A) A 10-0 suture attached to a long-armed needle is passed from the proximal iris tissue defect and the needle is threaded into the barrel of 26/30-gauge needle introduced from the opposite side that engages the distal iris tissue that is to be apposed. This is the railroad technique. (B) The suture loop is withdrawn from anterior chamber. (C) Four throws are taken through the loop. (D) Both the suture ends are pulled and the iris defect is narrowed down to a great extent. The suture ends are then cut with microscissors. (Republished with permission of Elsevier, from Narang P, Agarwal A, Agarwal A, Agarwal A. Twofold technique of nonappositional repair with single-pass four-throw pupilloplasty for iridodialysis. *J Cataract Refract Surg*, 44[12];2018; permission conveyed through Copyright Clearance Center, Inc.)

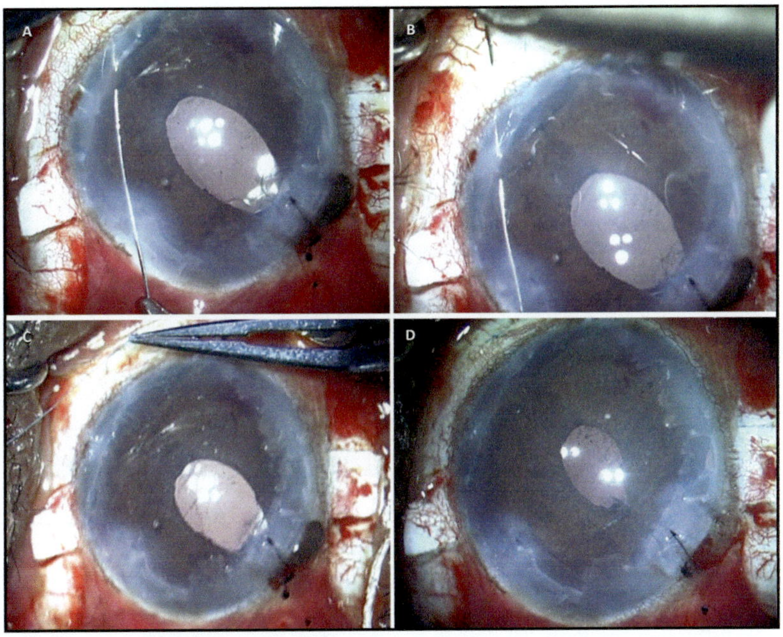

Figure 10-20. Part 2: Twofold technique for moderate to minimal iridodialysis. (A) A non-appositional repair is being performed and a 10-0 long-armed needle is passed from the paracentesis incision in a way that it engages the peripheral iris tissue that needs to be apposed. (B) The needle is withdrawn from the scleral side. (C) The second arm of the suture is passed through the adjacent iris tissue and the needle exits the eye on the scleral side. Both suture ends are tied. (D) The knot is formed and then buried in the scleral wall. (Republished with permission of Elsevier, from Narang P, Agarwal A, Agarwal A, Agarwal A. Twofold technique of nonappositional repair with single-pass four-throw pupilloplasty for iridodialysis. *J Cataract Refract Surg*, 44[12];2018; permission conveyed through Copyright Clearance Center, Inc.)

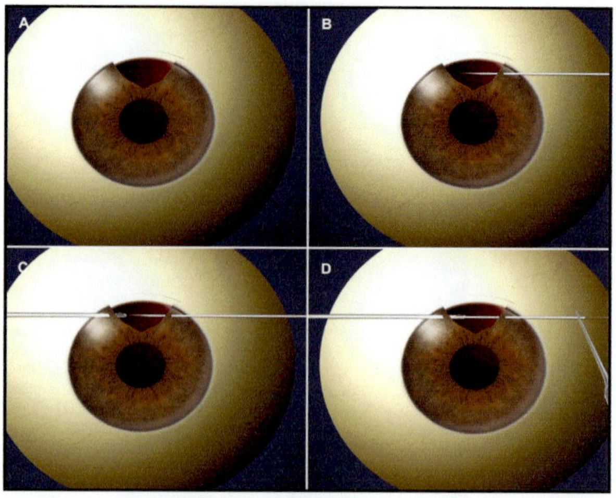

Figure 10-21. Part 1: Illustration of twofold technique for moderate to minimal iridodialysis. (A) A case of minimal iridodialysis. (B) A 10-0 suture attached to a long-armed needle is passed through the iris defect. (C) The needle is threaded into the barrel of a 26/30-gauge needle introduced from the opposite side that engages the distal iris tissue that is to be apposed. (D) This is the railroad technique.

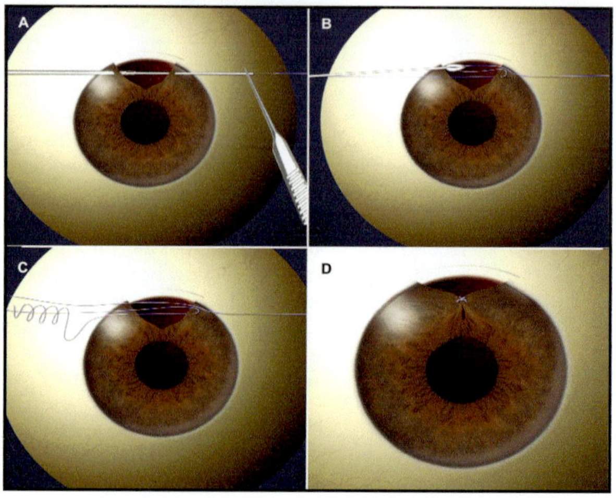

Figure 10-22. Part 2: Illustration of twofold technique for moderate to minimal iridodialysis. (A) Railroad technique completed. (B) The suture loop is withdrawn from the anterior chamber. (C) Four throws are taken through the loop. (D) Both the suture ends are pulled and the iris defect is narrowed down substantially. The suture ends are then cut with microscissors.

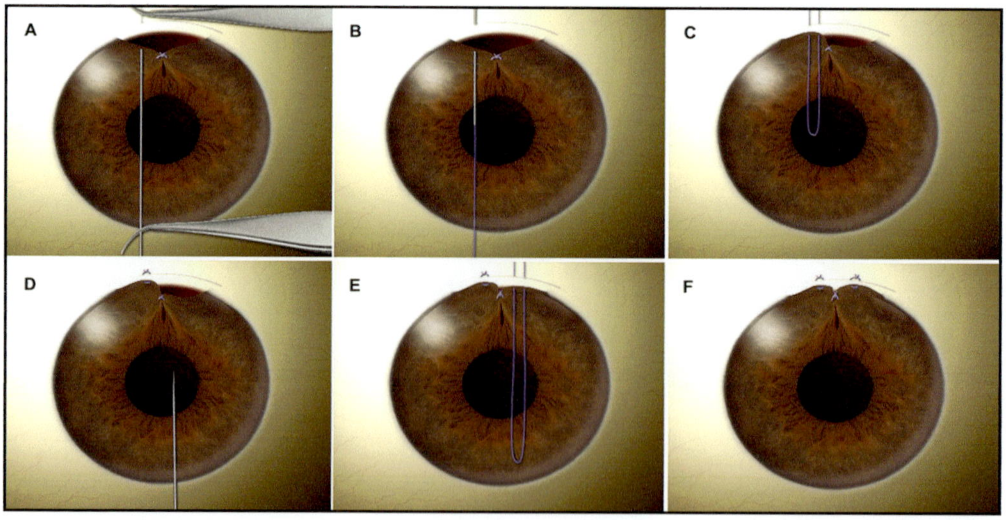

Figure 10-23. Part 3: Illustration of twofold technique for moderate to minimal iridodialysis. (A) The double-armed 10-0 polypropylene suture attached to a long-armed needle is passed through the peripheral iris tissue via a paracentesis. (B) The needle is brought out through a scleral groove. (C) The suture is brought out through the sclera and the other arm of the double-needle is also passed the same way. (D) The 2 ends of the suture are tied. The hang-back technique is repeated on the other side. (E) Hang-back technique. (F) Suture tied and the pupil restored.

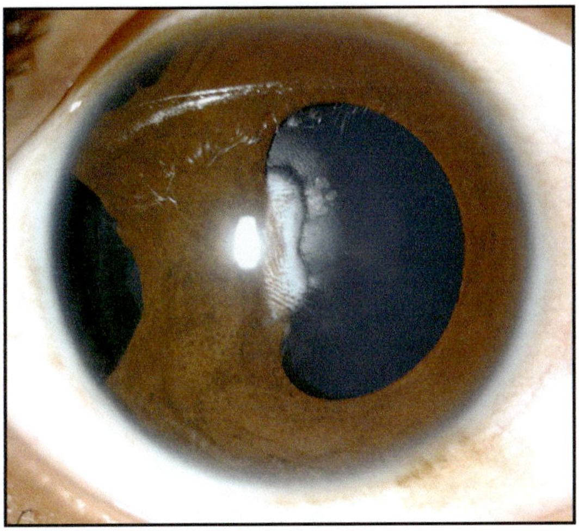

Figure 10-24. Minimal iridodialysis.

Discussion

Iridodialysis repair is an essential component to restore the architecture and integrity of the iris tissue (Figure 10-24). The twofold technique includes of all the advantages of the non-appositional technique and the SFT technique. The advantage of the non-appositional technique is not damaging the trabecular meshwork because the iris tissue does not cover the anterior chamber angle. This avoids the possibility of developing a secondary angle closure. SFT has the presumed advantage of inducing less inflammation and less pigment dispersion because it avoids unnecessary intervention in the anterior chamber. To summarize, the twofold technique facilitates iridodialysis repair and allows for correction of corectopia, thereby preventing glare and photophobia.

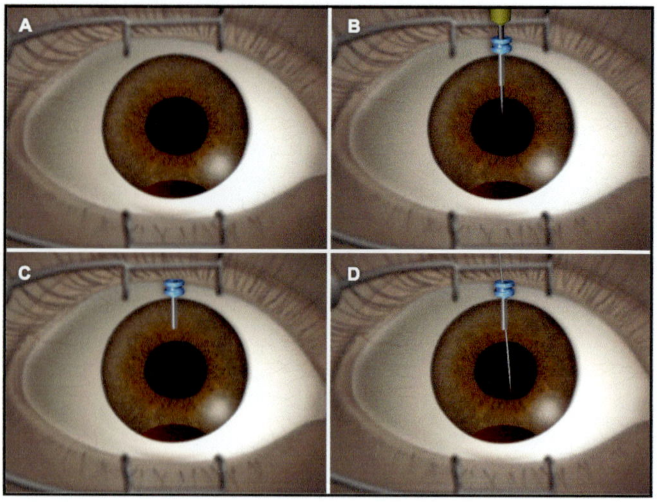

Figure 10-25. Part 1: Illustration of trocar-assisted hang-back technique. (A) Case demonstrating iridodialysis. (B) A 25-gauge trocar is introduced from the limbus from the opposite quadrant. (C) The trocar blade is withdrawn and the cannula is snugly fit. (D) A 10-0 polypropylene suture attached to the long-armed needle and is introduced from the lumen of the cannula.

Trocar-Assisted Non-Appositional Repair

During the iris repair maneuver, incorporation of corneal tissue into the suture needle leads to non-sliding of suture inside the eye. In order to overcome this aspect, trocar-assisted repair is proposed for performing an iridodialysis repair with non-appositional method. A 25-gauge trocar is placed inside the eye that is introduced from the limbus in the quadrant opposite to the area of iridodialysis. The 9-0 suture needle is passed through the trocar followed by engagement of the peripheral disinserted iris tissue. A 30-gauge needle is introduced from the scleral side and the suture needle is threaded into it and withdrawn from the eye. The second arm of the suture is again passed in the similar way engaging the area of adjacent iris tissue to the previous pass. Once both the suture needles are withdrawn, the loop of suture is pulled on the scleral side and a knot is tied and buried inside the scleral wall (Figures 10-25 through 10-27).

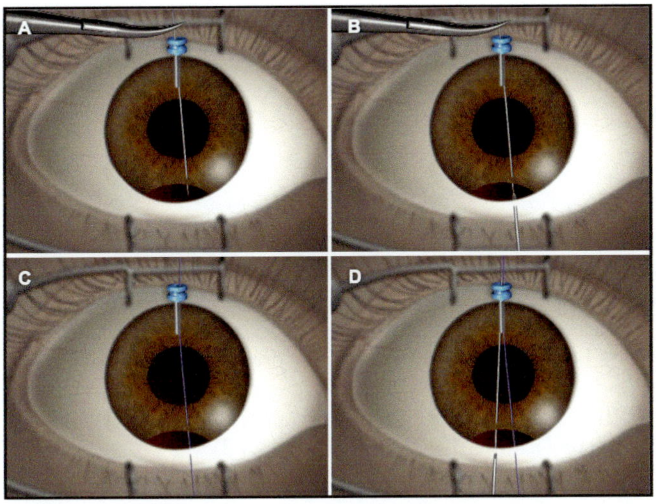

Figure 10-26. Part 2: Illustration of trocar-assisted hang-back technique. (A)The suture needle engages the rim of the peripheral iris tissue. (B) A 30-gauge needle is introduced from the scleral side and the suture needle is threaded into the barrel of the needle. (C) The 30-gauge needle that eventually pulls the suture along with it is withdrawn. (D) The second arm of the double-needle suture is similarly passed through the cannula and engages the iris rim adjacent to the previous pass. The suture is again threaded into the 30-gauge needle.

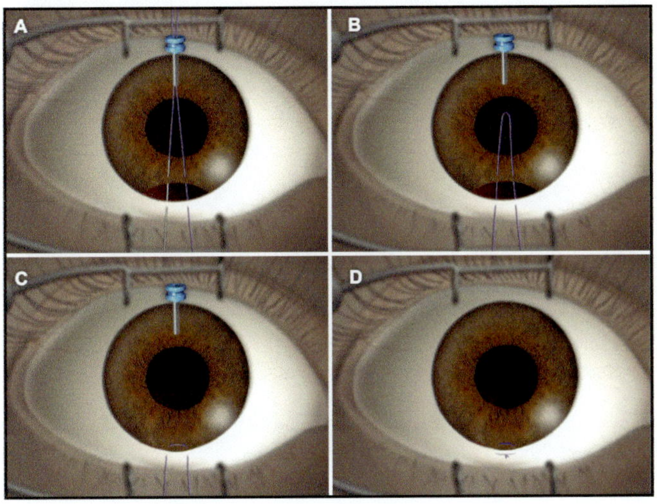

Figure 10-27. Part 3: Illustrated description of trocar-assisted hang-back technique. (A) The suture needle passes through the sclera. (B) Both suture ends are pulled. (C) The suture engages the peripheral iris tissue and it lies in close approximation to its insertion. (D) Both the suture ends are tied and a knot is formed.

Case Presentation 1

Twofold Technique for Iridodialysis Repair

Priya Narang, MS; Ashvin Agarwal, MBBS, MS; and Amar Agarwal, MS, FRCS, FRCOphth

During cataract surgery, a patient has an intraoperative complication. A posterior capsular rupture is noted in the initial phase of cataract surgery with non-emulsified nuclear fragments present in the anterior chamber. Two partial-thickness scleral flaps are made 180 degrees opposite each other, and sclerotomy is made about 1 mm away from the limbus, beneath the scleral flaps. The tip of the needle hits the iris base and iridodialysis is created. A 3-piece IOL is injected inside the anterior chamber and an IOL scaffold procedure is performed. After the nucleus is emulsified the same 3-piece IOL is fixed with the glued IOL procedure. The twofold technique is performed for iridodialysis repair (Figure 10-28 and Video 10-2).

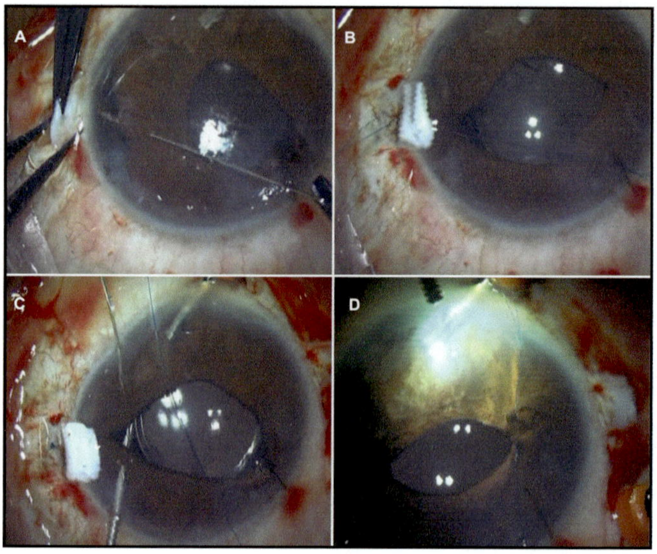

Figure 10-28. Twofold iridodialysis repair in a case of iatrogenic trauma. (A) Iatrogenic iridodialysis is observed during the stage of sclerotomy for glued secondary IOL fixation. A double-armed 10-0 suture needle is passed from the peripheral margin of the iris tissue and the needle is passed on to scleral surface. (B) Both ends of the double-armed suture are passed and pulled through the scleral side. (C) The SFT procedure is performed to correct corectopia induced due to overpull of the iris tissue during non-appositional repair. (D) Pupil reconstruction is complete.

Case Presentation 2

Iridodialysis Handled With Riveting Technique With Double-Flanged Polypropylene Suture

Mami Kusaka, MD and Masayuki Akimoto, MD, PhD

A patient presented with a cataract and traumatic iridodialysis that extended up to 90 degrees. The plan was to perform iridodialysis repair followed by cataract removal and IOL implantation.

Technique

The riveting technique was inspired by the Yamane method of intrascleral fixation of the IOL. A 6-0 Prolene (polypropylene) suture is held in close proximity of low temperature cautery so that it forms a bulb or a flange as in the Yamane technique. The heat causes the suture to shrink and eventually leads to the flange formation. The flange is then pressed and flattened (Figure 10-29 and Video 10-3).

A 30- or 27-gauge needle is passed from the iridodialysis area from the anterior chamber, and the 6-0 suture with the flange is threaded into it. The needle is then pulled out from the anterior chamber. The suture end is then pulled and the suture bulb holds the iris tissue against the scleral wall. The free end of suture is again heated with a low temperature cautery and the flange formed is buried in close proximity to the scleral wall as in Yamane technique.

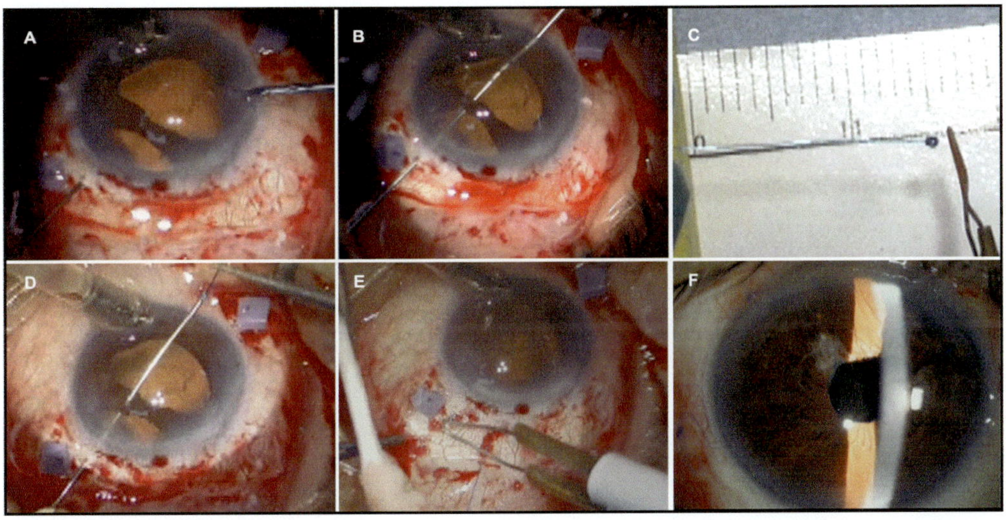

Figure 10-29. Iridodialysis handled with riveting technique with double-flanged polypropylene suture. (A) Iridodialysis. (B) Straight needle passed through sclera and iridodialysis. (C) Flange created with heating of a 6-0 Prolene suture. (D) Suture passed onto the needle. (E) Flange created at the scleral end. (F) Iridodialysis repaired.

References

1. Agarwal T, Singh D, Panda A. Guide needle-assisted iridodialysis repair [letter]. *J Cataract Refract Surg.* 2011;37:1918; reply by ME Snyder, LB Lindsell, 1918-1919.
2. Bardak Y, Ozerturk Y, Durmus M, Mensiz E, Aytuluner E. Closed chamber iridodialysis repair using a needle with a distal hole. *J Cataract Refract Surg.* 2000;26:173-176
3. Bhende P. Closed chamber iridodialysis repair using a needle with a distal hole. *J Cataract Refract Surg.* 2000; 26:1267-1268
4. Daglioglu MC, Coskun M, Ilhan N, Ayintap E, Tuzcu EA, Ilhan O, Oksuz H. Repair of iridodialysis using 8-0 polypropylene. *Semin Ophthalmol.* 2014;29:159-162
5. Khokhar S, Gupta S, Kumar G. Iridodialysis repair: stroke and dock technique. *Int Ophthalmol.* 2014;34:331-335
6. Snyder ME, Lindsell LB. Nonappositional repair of iridodialysis. *J Cataract Refract Surg.* 2011;37:625-628.
7. Voykov B. Knotless technique for iridodialysis repair. *Clin Experiment Ophthalmol.* 2016;44(2):135-136.
8. Wachler BB, Krueger RR. Double-armed McCannell suture for repair of traumatic iridodialysis. *Am J Ophthalmol.* 1996;122:109-110.
9. Narang P, Agarwal A, Agarwal A, Agarwal A. Twofold technique of nonappositional repair with single-pass four-throw pupilloplasty for iridodialysis. *J Cataract Refract Surg.* 2018;44(12):1413-1420.
10. Narang P, Agarwal A. Single-pass four-throw technique for pupilloplasty. *Eur J Ophthalmol.* 2017;27(4):506-508.

Please visit www.routledge.com/9781630917265

to access additional material.

11

Complications of Iris Repair and Pupilloplasty Techniques

Ashvin Agarwal, MBBS, MS; Priya Narang, MS; and Amar Agarwal, MS, FRCS, FRCOphth

Keywords

complications, iris reconstruction, pupilloplasty, single-pass four-throw pupilloplasty

Complications are an inherent part of any surgical maneuver. Surgeons should have adequate knowledge and technical skill to apprehend and tackle these challenging scenarios (Videos 11-1 and 11-2) in order to gain better results and promote safer surgery. Prevention is better than cure. The complications discussed are common to any type or method of pupilloplasty adopted by the surgeon.[1-10]

Prevention

Complications are inevitable, but the following are a few points to keep in mind to help prevent them and to make you a safer and more confident surgeon.

- Understanding stretching and pulling of iris tissue: When the iris tissue is held, it can behave very differently depending on the health of the tissue. For example, an atrophic tissue (Figure 11-1) will be friable, and a chaffed tissue will tear. Gauging the flexibility of iris tissue helps to understand the pull that the tissue can bear and withstand in the intraoperative and postoperative period.
- Taking the bite and engaging the iris tissue: When performing iris surgery, the most common step is to pass the needle through the iris tissue. When passing the needle for

Agarwal A, Agarwal A, eds. *Mastering Iris Repair: A Video Textbook of Iris Repair and Pupilloplasty Techniques* (pp 117-126).

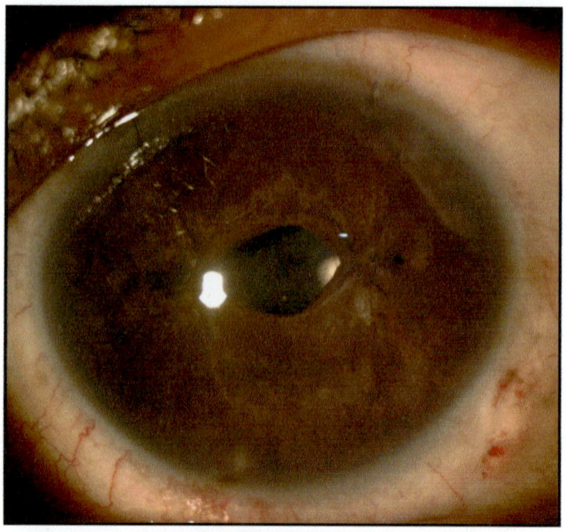

Figure 11-1. Note the patches of iris atrophy.

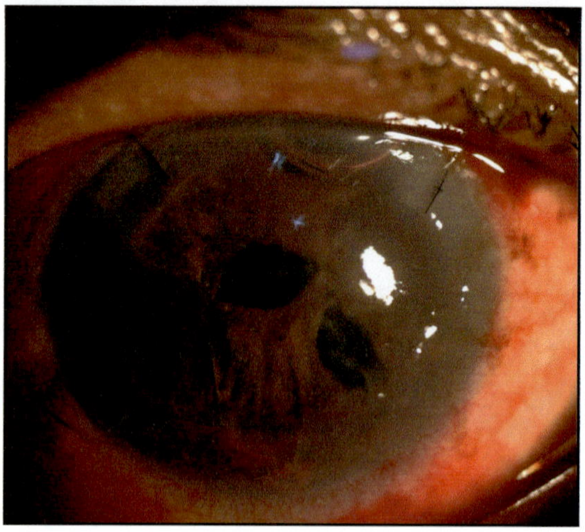

Figure 11-2. Tethering of the iris tissue is visible. Hyphema is also present in the anterior chamber.

a pupilloplasty technique, ensure that the needle does not pass too close to the pupillary margin; this prevents any tethering (Figure 11-2) or cheesewiring that might occur during the pulling maneuvers of this technique. For iridodialysis repair, ensure that the needle passes as close as possible to the iris root, as that is the portion of the iris that needs to be attached. This also helps leave enough iris tissue to construct the pupil at the end, preventing corectopia.

- Neovascular conditions: The surgeon should be cautious of neovascular conditions because they can lead to bleeding. Touching or handling such tissue could cause hyphema and its related complications.
- Medical history: Ask patients about their medical history, including if they take aspirin or blood thinners. These cases can be susceptible to intraoperative hyphema (see Figures 11-2 through 11-4). In planned cases, surgeons should check the bleeding and clotting time of their patients. Male patients should also be evaluated for history of medications for prostate disorders. In these cases, the iris tissue is floppy and behaves differently than the iris tissue of patients who do not take these drugs.

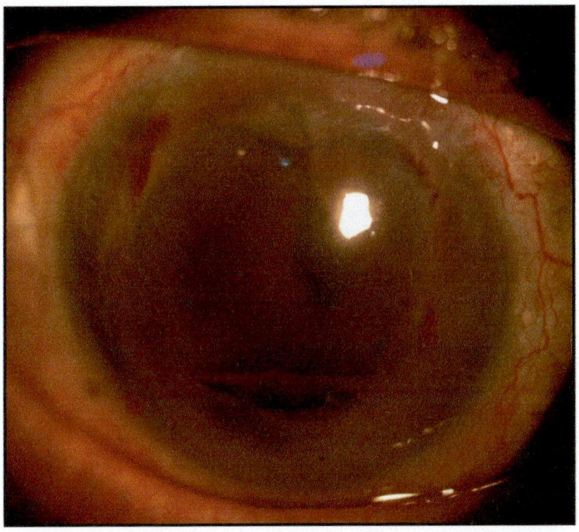

Figure 11-3. Total hyphema that obliterates the intraocular view.

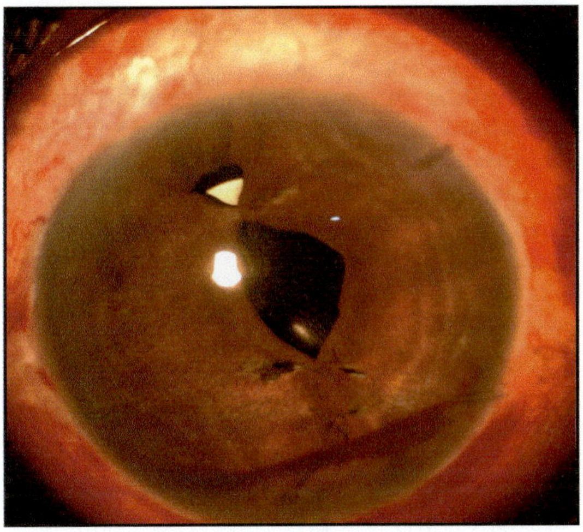

Figure 11-4. Blood clot formed in the anterior chamber.

Complications and Limitations

- Functional change of iris tissue: When performing an iris repair, we must keep in mind that any manipulation of the iris tissue affects its functional aspect, including the examination of pupillary reaction in neurological cases where it is essential to rule out afferent and efferent nerve defects.
- Hyphema: While performing an iris repair procedure, an intraoperative hyphema most commonly occurs when the root of the iris is inadvertently pulled and tears. This causes the blood vessels of the root to bleed profusely. This bleeding is often associated with increased intraocular pressure and, in prolonged cases, can lead to corneal staining. A hyphema often occurs when a small trickle of bleeding continues in the immediate postoperative period and slowly translates into total hyphema (see Figure 11-3).

  Hyphema can be graded as the following:

  0—Microhyphema (cells seen) but no visible layering

  1—Less than one-third of the anterior chamber filled with blood

  2—Blood fills one-third to half of the anterior chamber

  3—Blood fills half to two-thirds of the anterior chamber

  4—Blood fills the entire anterior chamber

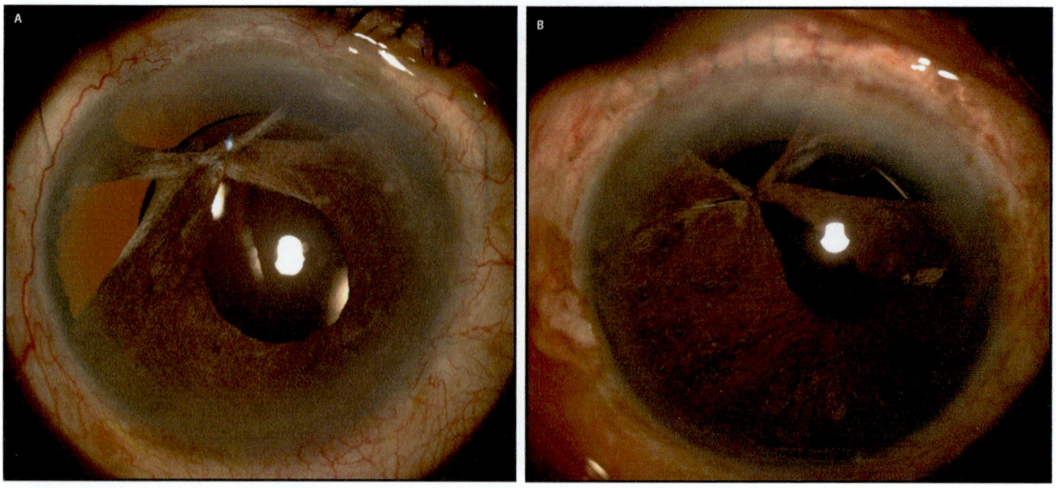

Figure 11-5. Iatrogenic iridodialysis.

- Management

  An anterior chamber wash is not helpful in handling an intraoperative bleed because it causes more bleeding. Instead, fill the anterior chamber with high-density viscoelastic to achieve an overfill for at least 2 to 5 minutes. Initially, this can be the right step in managing an intraoperative bleed because it helps to achieve an adequate tamponade.

  If the blood in the anterior chamber clots, then the clot can be easily pulled out of the eye (see Figure 11-4). These patients can be administered an oral dose of serratiopeptidase enzyme that helps to resolve the blood. The intraocular pressure should be monitored and measures should be taken to keep it in check in the postoperative period.

- Iridodialysis: Iridodialysis is a common complication during iris repair, especially with novice surgeons. As the suture needle passes through the iris on both sides, control of the needle is sometimes lost, leading to inadvertent movements that pull and tear the iris from its root, causing iridodialysis. The most common cause of inducing an iatrogenic iridodialysis is due to the surgeon taking a large bite of iris tissue and then, while apposing the proximal and distal parts of iris, pulling up to such an extent that the iris root gives way and iridodialysis occurs (Figure 11-5). For tips on management of iridodialysis, please refer to Chapter 6.
- Corectopia: At times, over- or undercorrection lead to eccentric pupils that are not in the visual axis and cause visual disturbances. Corectopia occurs due to unequal involvement of iris tissue in the suture needle that tends to pull it eccentrically (Figure 11-6). The management of this condition should be considered on a case-by-case basis. Sometimes doing less for the patient is best because additional interventions may weaken the iris and cause it to tear more, leaving it more friable, with gapes and holes. Corectopia with minimal or no visual disturbances should be left in situ without any further interventions (Figure 11-7). Surgeons can attempt a pupillary correction of the pupil border in the area of updrawn pupil in cases with functional disturbances.
- Polycoria: This unwanted scenario is encountered when the iris tissue gapes and is friable. This situation is often encountered in traumatic cases that have massive iris involvement, such as iris prolapse or total iris disinsertion. Multiple pupils are seen that are iatrogenic (Figure 11-8).
- Transillumination defects: These defects are seen in overtly thin iris tissue due to either overstretching or an inherently thin iris. They usually do not pose any problems in the postoperative period. The iris tissue often becomes thin and atrophic due to overt manipulations in the anterior chamber such as frequent rubbing of the iris that releases iris pigments.

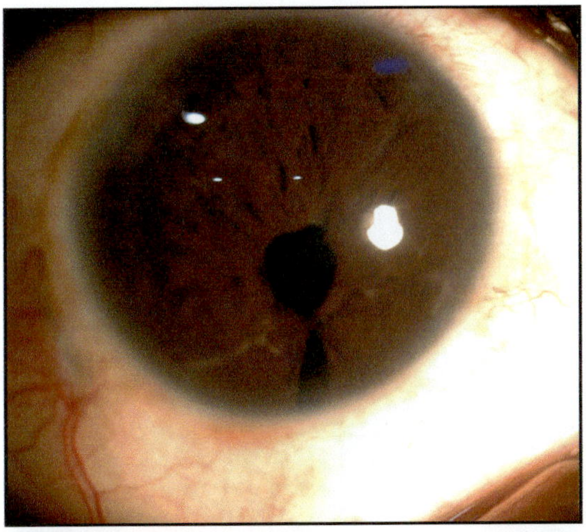

Figure 11-6. Corectopia with massively eccentric pupil.

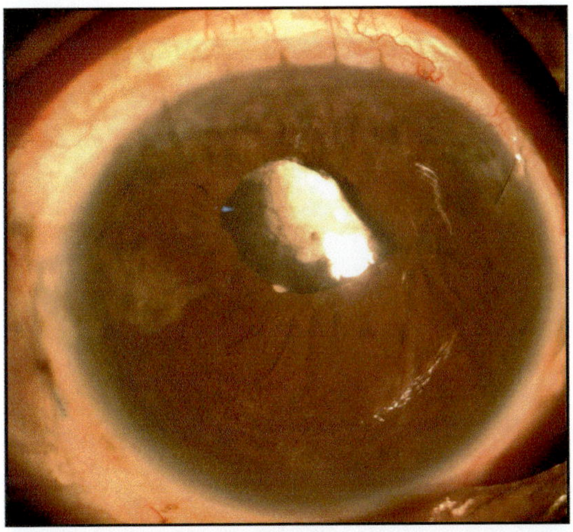

Figure 11-7. Mild corectopia.

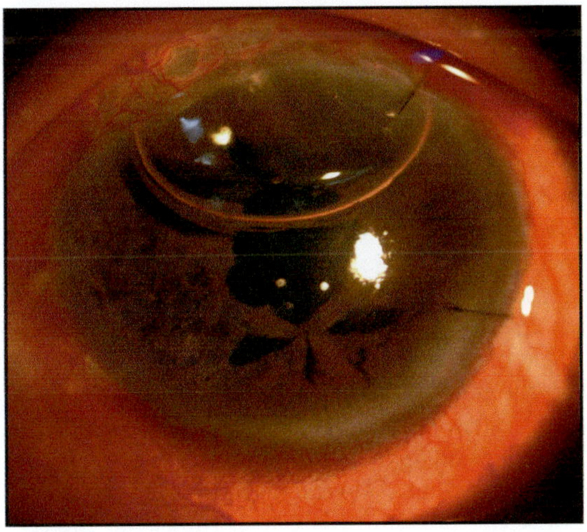

Figure 11-8. Polycoria.

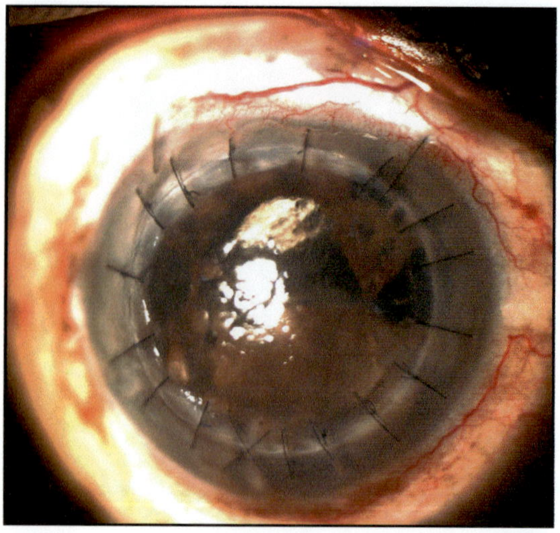

Figure 11-9. Tethering of the iris tissue.

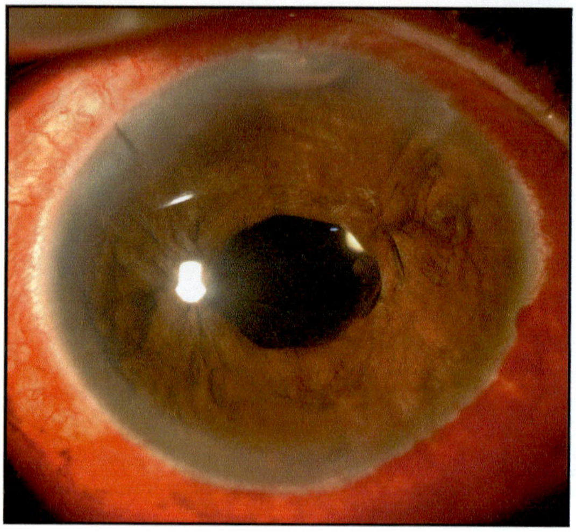

Figure 11-10. Fibrin membrane on the intraocular lens (IOL).

- Tethering or cheesewiring of iris tissue: This occurs when the suture bite is too close to the pupil margin. The stretch forces make the iris tissue give way causing cheesewiring (Figure 11-9). When the needle passes through the atrophic patch, cheesewiring occurs because the atrophic patch cannot hold the stress of the iris tissue pull.
- Fibrin membrane and exudates and pigment dispersion: Overt handling of the iris tissue leads to an increased postoperative inflammatory response that causes fibrin membrane formation, which can be thin or thick (Figure 11-10). Exudate and pigment deposits on the IOL surface are an indicator of prior inflammation (Figure 11-11). Increased manipulation and pronounced inflammatory response often also lead to corneal edema (Figure 11-12). These cases can be managed with a tapered dose of topical steroids and anti-inflammatory drugs. Cycloplegics are often advised to reduce the pain and postoperative inflammation.
- Non-dilating pupil: Performing pupilloplasty narrows down the pupillary aperture, which can make future interventions in the posterior segment difficult (Figure 11-13). Postoperatively, the pupil does not dilate to a great extent. However, the single-pass four-throw technique has been demonstrated to allow the pupil to dilate to 3 times the surface area, providing adequate posterior segment visualization.[11]

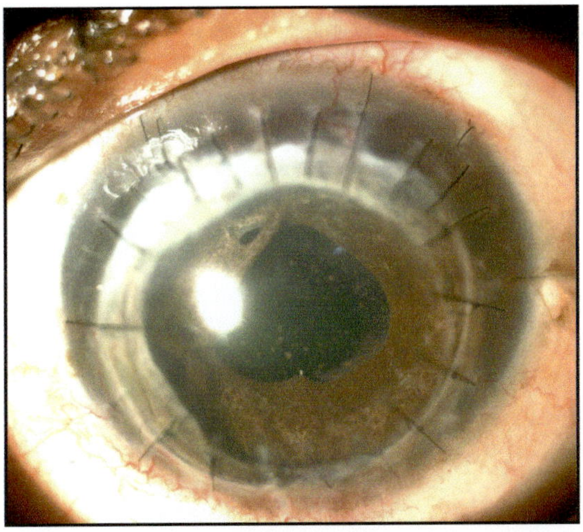

Figure 11-11. Pigment dispersion on the IOL.

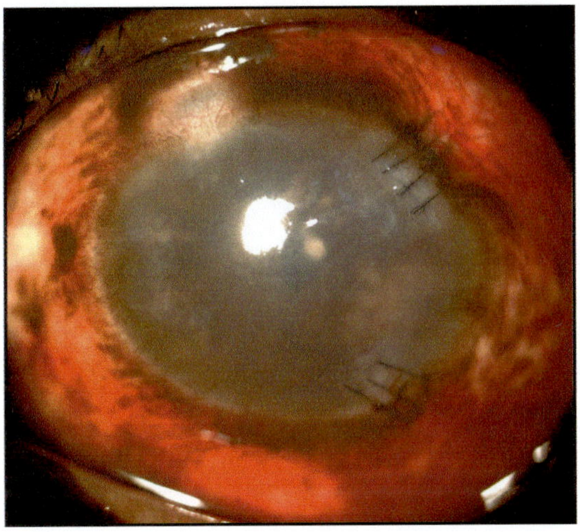

Figure 11-12. Corneal edema due to a massive inflammatory response.

- Non-sliding of the suture loop in the anterior chamber: This situation is encountered when the suture needle involves a part of the corneal tissue that prevents the loop from sliding inside the anterior chamber when both the suture ends are pulled. Excessive pulling does not slide the loop internally. On the contrary, it leads to cheesewiring of the iris tissue in the other quadrant. At this juncture, the surgeon should cut the suture and re-do the pupilloplasty procedure.

Discussion

Although there many complications that can be associated with the pupilloplasty procedure, the benefits of performing the procedure outweigh them because of the functional and cosmetic benefits to the patient. Delicately and appropriately handling the tissue prevents many unexpected outcomes and optimizes the surgical output.

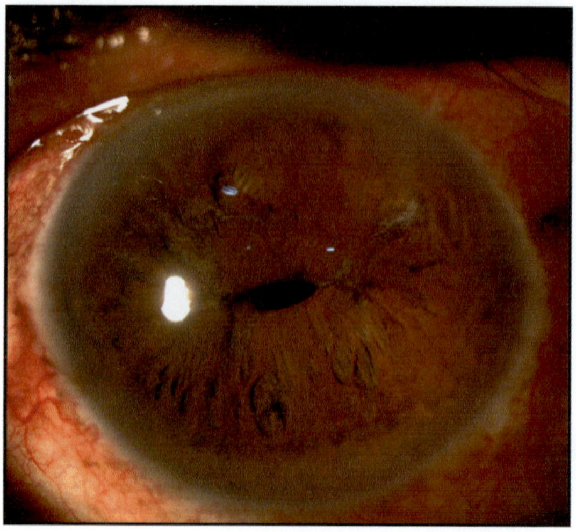

Figure 11-13. Pupillary phimosis and non-dilating pupil following a surgical pupilloplasty.

Case Presentation

Iatrogenic Iridodialysis Complication and Management

Ashvin Agarwal, MBBS, MS; Priya Narang, MS; and
Amar Agarwal, MS, FRCS, FRCOphth

A case of a 1-piece foldable subluxated IOL that had to be repaired. A glued IOL was planned with a 3-piece IOL. A scleral tunnel incision was made to explant the subluxated IOL. While performing the sclerotomy for the glued IOL, an inadvertent iridodialysis was created.

Glued intrascleral fixation of an IOL is an established procedure for IOL fixation in eyes with deficient posterior capsule. The advantage of the glued IOL technique is the absence of pseudophacodonesis, as detected on high frame per second recording, which automatically translates into better postoperative visual outcomes. The technique's shortcoming is the absence of specially designed IOLs that can be implanted in eyes with greater white-to-white diameter. In such a scenario, anterior sclerotomy is often performed that shifts the plane of the IOL anteriorly, allowing for more haptic externalization. During this endeavor, the peripheral iris often gets entrapped into the needle that is employed for sclerotomy resulting in iridodialysis, hyphema and, occasionally, an iris tear or an accidental creation of a sclerotomy channel that is anterior to the iris plane. To avert this complication, peripheral iridectomy is performed in eyes with greater white-to-white diameter undergoing the glued IOL procedure. A vitrector-assisted peripheral iridectomy allows for appropriate and adequate access to the peripheral iris tissue that can be cut in a controlled manner. Lowering the cuts per minute of the vitrector allows for adequate time for the iris tissue to get engaged in the mouth of the vitrector. If a surgeon performs peripheral iridectomy at a high cuts per minute, then there is a chance of extra engagement of the iris tissue into the vitrector that can eventually lead to big peripheral iridectomy or a complete sectoral iridectomy. Performing a peripheral iridectomy also facilitates smooth entry and exit of glued IOL forceps from the sclerotomy site and allows haptic externalization without any hindrance. Therefore, performing a peripheral iridectomy helps to avert iris-related complications in the glued IOL procedure.

After the iridodialysis occurred, the superior iris prolapsed and had to be repaired as well. A single-pass four-throw pupilloplasty was performed for the superior iris prolapse. Then a hang-back technique was performed using double-armed 9-0 Prolene (Ethicon) sutures for the iridodialysis (Figure 11-14 and Video 11-3).

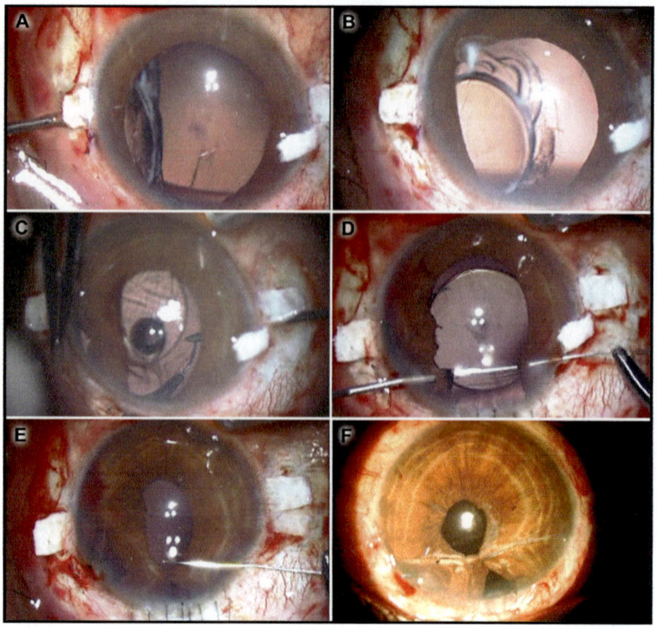

Figure 11-14. Iatrogenic iridodialysis management. (A) Subluxated 1-piece foldable posterior chamber IOL. (B) Vitrectomy is performed and the IOL explanted through a scleral tunnel incision. (C) Inadvertent iridodialysis seen while performing the anterior sclerotomy with a 22-gauge needle. (D) Single-pass four-throw pupilloplasty for superior iris prolapse. (E) Hang-back technique for the iridodialysis using a double-armed Prolene suture. (F) Postoperative picture shows a glued IOL with iris repair. Vision is 20/20.

References

1. Siepser SB. The closed-chamber slipping suture technique for iris repair. *Ann Ophthalmol.* 1994;26:71-72.
2. Osher RH, Snyder ME, Cionni RJ. Modification of the Siepser slip-knot technique. *J Cataract Refract Surg.* 2005;31:1098-1100.
3. Snyder ME, Osher RH. Techniques and principles of surgical management of the traumatic cataract. In: Steinert RF, ed. *Cataract Surgery: Techniques, Complications and Management.* 2nd ed. Philadelphia, PA: Saunders;2004:331-329.
4. Chang DF. Siepser slipknot for McCannel iris-suture fixation of subluxated intraocular lenses. *J Cataract Refract Surg.* 2004;30:1170-1176.
5. McCannel MA. A retrievable suture idea for anterior uveal problems. *Ophthalmic Surg.* 1976;7:98-103.
6. Ogawa GSH. The iris cerclage suture for permanent mydriasis: a running suture technique. *Ophthalmic Surg Lasers.* 1998;29:1001-1009.
7. Wachler BBS, Krueger RR. Double-armed McCannel suture for repair of traumatic iridodialysis. *Am J Ophthalmol.* 1996;122:109-110.
8. Kaufman SC, Insler MS. Surgical repair of a traumatic iridodialysis. *Ophthalmic Surg Lasers.* 1996;27:963-966.
9. Schoenberg ED, Price FW Jr. Modification of Siepser sliding suture technique for iris repair and endothelial keratoplasty. *J Cataract Refract Surg.* 2014;40:705-708.
10. Narang P, Agarwal A. Single-pass four-throw technique for pupilloplasty. *Eur J Ophthalmol.* 2017;27:506-508.
11. Kumar DA, Agarwal A, Srinivasan M, Narendrakumar J, Mohanavelu A, Krishnakumar A. Single pass four throw (SFT) pupilloplasty: postoperative mydriasis and fundus visibility in pseudophakic eyes. *J Cataract Refract Surg.* 2017;43(10):1307-1312.

SECTION III

EXTENDED IMPLICATIONS OF IRIS AND PUPIL REPAIR

12

Aniridia

*Ashar Agarwal, MS, FRCS; Priya Narang, MS;
and Amar Agarwal, MS, FRCS, FRCOphth*

KEYWORDS

aniridia, coloboma, congenital abnormalities of the iris, iris defect, iris deficiency

Aniridia is a clinical entity characterized by hypoplasia, or absence of iris tissue, that may be genetic, traumatic, or iatrogenic in origin.[1-11] The genetic origin is usually bilateral and is associated with other ocular defects (Figure 12-1). Congenital aniridia is rare and has an incidence of 1 per 50,000 to 100,000 live births. About two-thirds are familial. One-third occur without a family history from a new genetic mutation in the *PAX6* gene and have a 30% chance of developing Wilms' tumor. Serial renal ultrasound is required to rule out Wilms' tumor, especially in patients with no family history. Aniridia occurs as an autosomal dominant gene, inherited from a parent in two-thirds of cases and as a mutation in the *PAX6* gene in one-third of cases. Aniridia may occur sporadically, or as a chromosome deletion of the short arm of chromosome 11. It may also occur following trauma or as an intraoperative incident (Figure 12-2).

The genetic variant of aniridia may be associated with glaucoma. In the hereditary form, though the iris appears absent, gonioscopy does show the iris root. The trabecular meshwork may be partially or completely covered by the iris stump. An iris stump is generally visible. The trabecular meshwork may be normal, partly developed, or abnormal. Peripheral anterior synechiae may be observed.

Degree of visual impairment is not correlated with the degree of aniridia. Instead, it is generally because of other associated ocular conditions, such as cataract, corneal changes, glaucoma, optic nerve damage, and macular hypoplasia, all of which lead to decreased vision, nystagmus, strabismus, and amblyopia. Uncontrolled glaucoma can also cause visual loss over time. Photophobia and

Agarwal A, Agarwal A, eds. *Mastering Iris Repair: A Video Textbook of Iris Repair and Pupilloplasty Techniques* (pp 129-135).

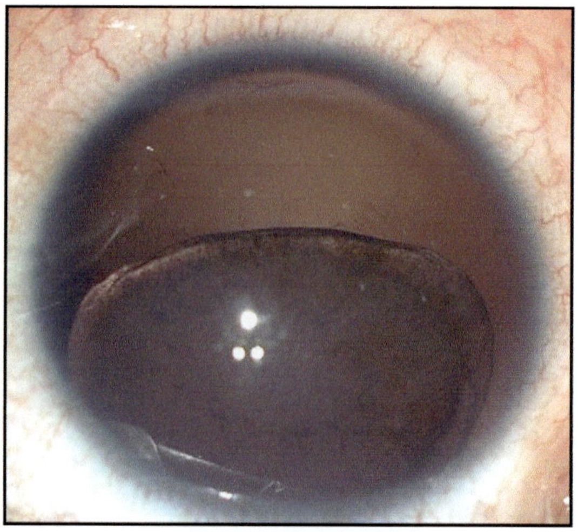

Figure 12-1. Congenital subluxated lens with aniridia.

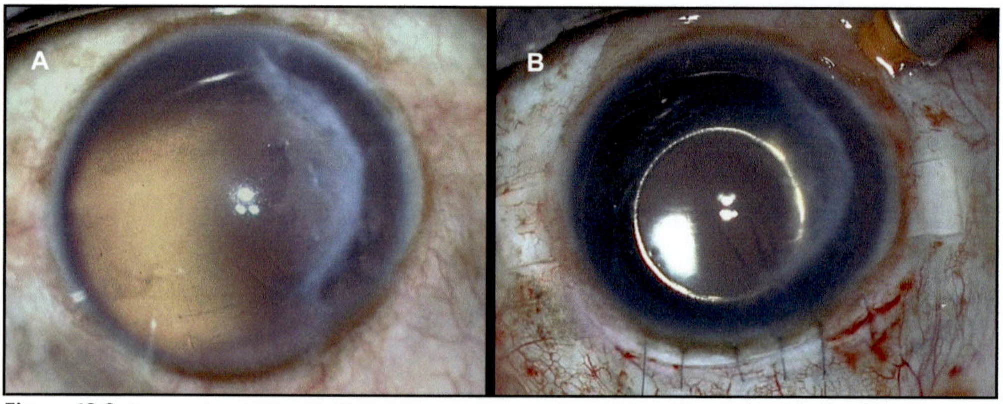

Figure 12-2. Traumatic aniridia. (A) Clinical image of traumatic aniridia with aphakia. (B) Glued iris prosthesis (aniridia glued intraocular lens [IOL]) implanted. Note the 23-gauge trocar cannula used as infusion.

decreased visual acuity are common symptoms. Limbal stem cell deficiency, pannus, microcornea, and ulcers may be present. About 50% to 85% of patients develop lens opacities in the first 2 decades of having the disease. Phacodonesis, ectopia lentis, and complete lens dislocation may occur.

Management

Glaucoma may be managed medically or surgically with a trabeculectomy, trabeculotomy, or goniotomy. Care should be taken to avoid damage to the crystalline lens, zonules, and the vitreous during glaucoma surgery. Endocyclophotocoagulation and tube shunts are rarely needed. Photophobia and nystagmus may be managed with special contact lenses or IOLs. Any refractive error should be corrected, amblyopia treated, and strabismus surgery performed if indicated. Corneal pathology may require penetrating keratoplasty or Boston keratoprosthesis; however, potential complications secondary to associated limbal stem cell deficiency must be clearly kept in mind during decision making.

Coexistent cataract is often present and can be managed, depending on the case. Minimal cataracts and subluxations may be left alone. In the bag IOL implantation needs to be decided only after taking into consideration the increased risk of progressive zonular dialysis in these patients. Aniridia rings (Figures 12-3 through 12-5) may be used for creating an artificial iris. Aniridia IOL (Figure 12-6) may also be used for this purpose. Subluxated cataracts may be removed by

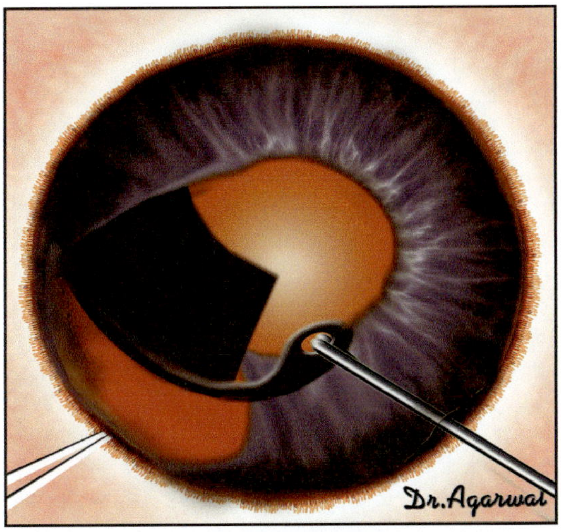

Figure 12-3. Coloboma shield capsular tension ring. Coloboma shields or aniridia segments have an integrated 60- to 90-degree tinted sector shield. The leading end is delivered into the capsular bag with McPherson forceps. The trailing end is dialed or inserted into the bag with micro–rhexis forceps. It is rotated so that the sector shield lies beneath the iris defect. (Reprinted with permission from Agarwal A, ed. *Illustrative Guide to Cataract Surgery: A Step-by-Step Approach to Refining Surgical Skills*. Thorofare, NJ: SLACK Incorporated; 2011.)

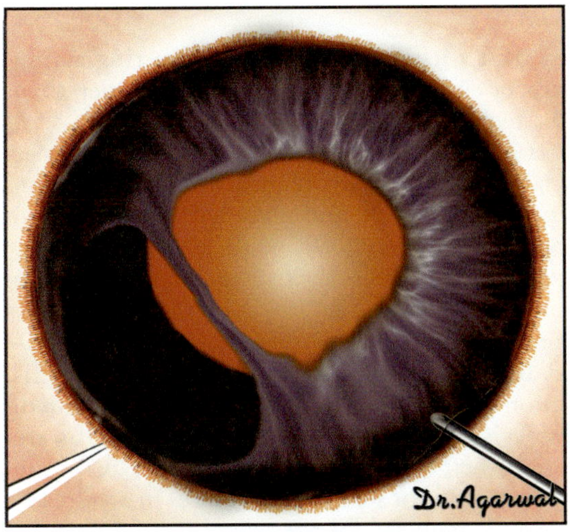

Figure 12-4. Coloboma shield capsular tension ring. The coloboma shields protect against glare and monocular diplopia. They can be used in patients with large sector iridectomies and traumatic iris defects. For defects greater than 90 degrees, 2 rings can be implanted with the sector shields placed adjacent to each other. (Reprinted with permission from Agarwal A, ed. *Illustrative Guide to Cataract Surgery: A Step-by-Step Approach to Refining Surgical Skills*. Thorofare, NJ: SLACK Incorporated; 2011.)

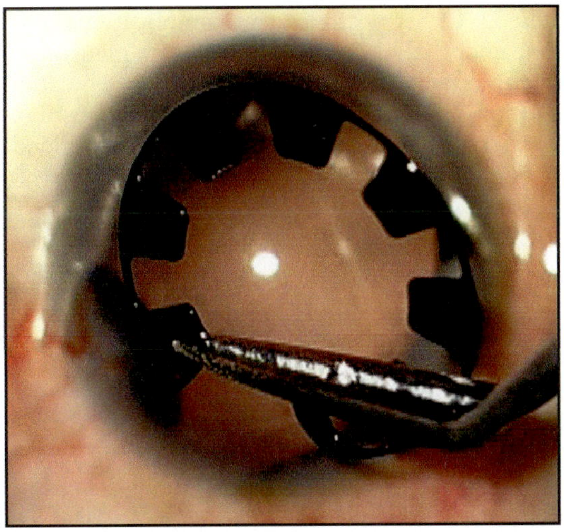

Figure 12-5. Aniridia with subluxated cataract. Multisegmented aniridia capsular tension ring come in pairs. Both are inserted into the bag and work like a venetian blind.

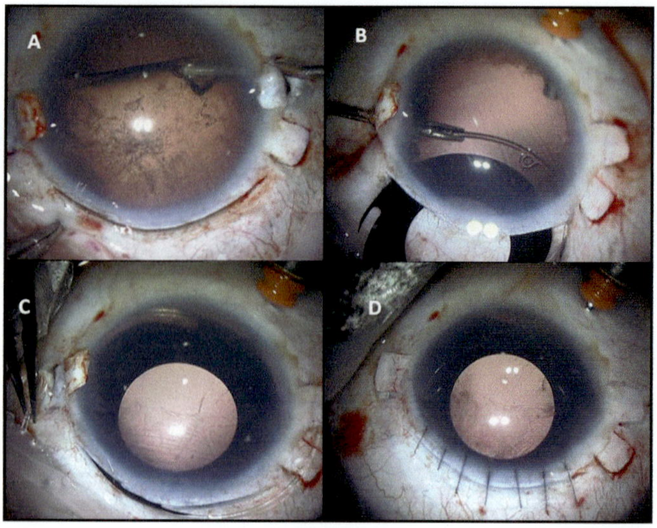

Figure 12-6. Glued aniridia IOL implantation. (A) Two scleral flaps made diagonally apart and lensectomy done via the sclerotomy. (B) Limbal incision made and aniridia IOL inserted through the wound. (C) IOL haptic externalized by the handshake method and tucked in scleral tunnels. (D) Limbal wound sutured and flaps apposed with fibrin glue.

lensectomy, and a glued aniridia IOL placed. These IOLs have a peripheral opaque ring acting as an artificial iris. These 1-piece polymethyl methacrylate lenses are larger and heavier than standard IOLs. For stability, we prefer a glued IOL technique to sclerally fixate these IOLs. A larger corneoscleral tunnel is required. Haptic exteriorization must be performed with care as the polymethyl methacrylate haptic may break. A larger sclerotomy is required. Another option in cataractous lenses is to retain the anterior and posterior capsule and place the aniridia glued IOL over the capsule. This gives additional support to the heavier IOL while also maintaining the vitreous phase intact. In children, a posterior curvilinear capsulorrhexis may be performed to avoid visual axis opacification.

In patients with congenital aniridia, limbal stem cell deficiency is often an associated feature.[9] Hence, a minimal conjunctival peritomy and an incision posterior to the limbal stem cells are preferred during surgery. Meticulous manipulation of scleral and limbal tissue is warranted. Intraoperative hyphema from damage to ciliary vessels is common when suture fixated IOLs are used;[11] however, this complication is not encountered when transscleral glued aniridia IOLs are used.[6,7] In case of traumatic aniridia, manipulation of the anterior segment structures in an already injured eye is particularly challenging. A larger incision is required for the scleral fixated aniridia IOLs that implies the risk of surgically induced astigmatism. A postoperative rise in intraocular pressure is the most common complication encountered.[6] Other postoperative complications that have been reported include persistent inflammation, endothelial cell loss, secondary glaucoma, macular edema, hypotony, and ciliochoroidal detachment.[11] The possibility of suture-related complications, like suture knot exposure, suture erosion, and disintegration leading to possible dislocation of the IOL, cannot be ignored with transscleral suture-fixated IOLs.[6] However, glued aniridia IOLs are free of this complication and show good IOL centration in the long term.

Acquired Aniridia

Aniridia may occur following trauma. This is generally associated with extensive ocular injury as in the case presented at the end of this chapter of pseudophacocele with total traumatic aniridia. Any associated vitreous pathology may require the assistance of a vitreoretinal surgeon. Iatrogenic aniridia may occur during phaco, especially if there is already coexistent iridodialysis or a very floppy iris. These cases are often complex and have other associated morbidities. In case of complete iris avulsion, an aniridia glued IOL may be used.

Aniridia Glued IOL

In eyes with aphakia and associated aniridia, aniridia IOL can be fixed in the eye with the glued IOL procedure. In eyes with a subluxated lens, a lensectomy is initially performed followed by glued aniridia IOL (see Figure 12-6). Two partial-thickness lamellar scleral flaps are made 180 degrees diagonally apart, sclerotomy is made 1 to 1.5 mm from the limbus, and the sclerocorneal incision for the IOL is made superiorly. Anterior vitrectomy is performed, and the IOL is inserted in the scleral tunnel. The haptics are externalized under the scleral flaps using the handshake technique and are then tucked into the intralamellar scleral tunnel (Scharioth pocket) created with a 26-gauge needle. Vitrectomy is performed at the sclerotomy site and the flaps are sealed with the application of fibrin glue on to the bed of the scleral flap (Video 12-1).

Discussion

The term *aniridia* is considered to be a misnomer because a small portion of iris tissue is always detected on gonioscopy. Patients with aniridia should be evaluated for refractory errors and ocular deviations, such as esotropia, which is encountered more often than any other tropias. Posterior segment evaluation should be performed for optic nerve or foveal hypoplasia that may be associated with nystagmus.

It is recommended that all patients with aniridia undergo an annual glaucoma screening. Measurement of intraocular pressure, examination of the angle for evidence of closure, optic disk examination, and visual field testing should be performed. Central corneal thickness should always be measured, as patients with aniridia have corneas up to 100 μm thicker than average, which can influence intraocular pressure readings.[11] Occasionally, hearing difficulties may be encountered in these patients.

Ocular management of cases with aniridia depends on the clinical scenario and complaints of the patient along with associated systemic abnormalities (see Video 12-1). Implantation of the modified capsular tension rings with occluder paddle and aniridia IOLs help solve the majority of cases. Nevertheless, the visual potential in aniridia cases is often limited due to the involvement of various structures of the eye.

Case Presentation

Iatrogenic Aniridia

Ashar Agarwal, MS, FRCS; Priya Narang, MS; and Amar Agarwal, MS, FRCS, FRCOphth

Figure 12-7 highlights a case of traumatic iridodialysis with subluxated lens. The patient reported a history of trauma with dimness of vision. Iris repair with removal of cataract was planned for the case. Intraoperatively, the iridodialysis portion is initially fixed and lens removal is started. During the course of the surgery, the iris tissue gets trapped in the phacoemulsification probe and total aniridia is witnessed. An aniridia IOL is then fixed for the case (Video 12-2).

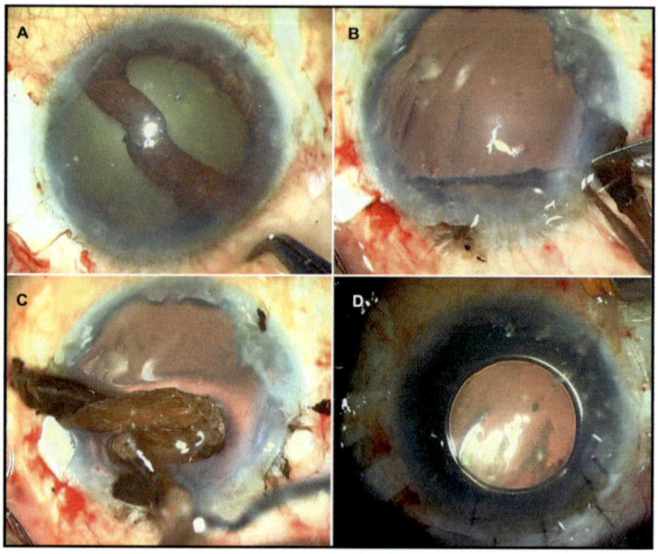

Figure 12-7. Clinical case of iridodialysis leading to iatrogenic aniridia. (A) Massive iridodialysis seen with subluxation of lens. (B) Iatrogenic iridodialysis. (C) Total iatrogenic aniridia. (D) Aniridia IOL fixed by the glued IOL technique.

References

1. Nelson LB, Spaeth GL, Nowinski TS, Margo CE, Jackson L. Aniridia: a review. *Surv Ophthalmol.* 1984;28:621-642.
2. Schneider S, Osher RH, Burk SE, Lutz TB, Montione R. Thinning of the anterior capsule associated with congenital aniridia. *J Cataract Refract Surg.* 2003;29:523-525.
3. Hou ZQ, Hao YS, Wang W, Ma ZZ, Zhong YF, Song SJ. Clinical pathological study of the anterior lens capsule abnormalities in familial congenital aniridia with cataract. *Beijing Da Xue Xue Bao.* 2005;37:494-497.
4. Pozdeyeva NA, Pashtayev NP, Lukin VP, Batkov YN. Artificial iris lens diaphragm in reconstructive surgery for aniridia and aphakia. *J Cataract Refract Surg.* 2005;31:1750-1759.
5. Choyce P. *Intraocular Lenses and Implants.* London, United Kingdom: HK Lewis. 1964.
6. Kumar, DA, Agarwal A, Jacob S, Lamba M, Packialakshmi S, Meduri A. Combined surgical management of capsular and iris deficiency with glued intraocular lens technique. *J Refract Surg.* 2013;29(5):342-347.
7. Kumar DA, Agarwal A, Prakash G, Jacob S. Managing total aniridia with aphakia using a glued iris prosthesis. *J Cataract Refract Surg.* 2010;36(5):864-865.
8. Burk SE, Da Mata AP, Snyder ME, Cionni RJ, Cohen JS, Osher RH. Prosthetic iris implantation for congenital, traumatic, or functional iris deficiencies. *J Cataract Refract Surg.* 2001;27:1732-1740.
9. Sundmacher T, Reinhard T, Althaus C. Black diaphragm intraocular lens in congenital aniridia. *Ger J Ophthalmol.* 1994;3:197-201.
10. Agarwal A, Jacob S, Kumar DA, Agarwal A, Narasimhan S, Agarwal A. Handshake technique for glued intrascleral haptic fixation of a posterior chamber intraocular lens. *J Cataract Refract Surg.* 2013;39(3):317-322
11. Lee H, Khan R, O'Keefe M. Aniridia: current pathology and management. *Acta Ophthalmologica.* 2008;86(7):708-715.

Please visit www.routledge.com/9781630917265

to access additional material.

13

Pinhole Pupilloplasty

Priya Narang, MS; Amar Agarwal, MS FRCS FRCOphth;
and Ashvin Agarwal, MBBS, MS

Keywords

pinhole pupilloplasty, pinhole, pupilloplasty, single-pass four-throw pupilloplasty, small aperture optics

The definition of pinhole pupilloplasty is self-explanatory as it states that a pinhole pupil can be achieved with the procedure of surgical pupilloplasty.[1] Technically, pupilloplasty is a procedure that is employed for pupil reconstruction to prevent glare and photophobia. Currently, surgical pupilloplasty has found an application in the refractive arena as well because decreasing the size of pupil has been found to improve visual and image quality.[1] The further application of pinhole pupilloplasty for achieving extended depth of focus is currently being investigated.

Principle of Pinhole Pupilloplasty

Pinhole visual acuity is the best possible vision that can be attained in a patient. Pinhole pupilloplasty works on the same principle as a pinhole that helps focus the central and paracentral rays in cases with higher order corneal aberrations. Pinhole pupilloplasty wards off the peripheral unfocused rays thereby enhancing the visual quality and image (Figure 13-1). It also works on the principle of the Stiles-Crawford effect (Figure 13-2), where the light entering the eye from the center of the pupil creates a greater photoreceptor response as compared to light entering from the peripheral edge of the pupil.[2,3] As the pinhole is created, only central rays are focused, creating a greater cone photoreceptor response (Video 13-1).

Agarwal A, Agarwal A, eds. *Mastering Iris Repair: A Video Textbook of Iris Repair and Pupilloplasty Techniques* (pp 137-144).

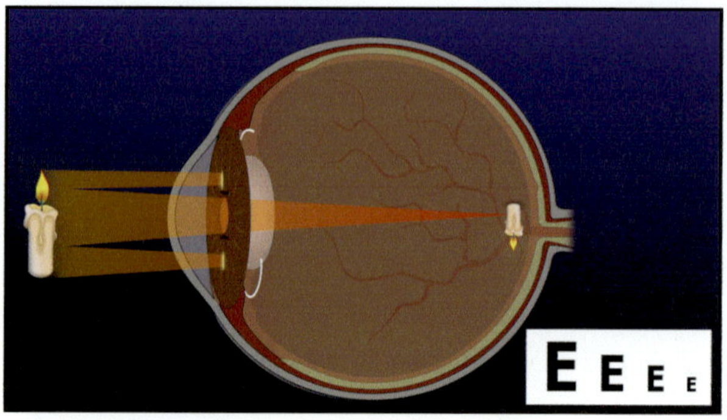

Figure 13-1. Image depicting the principle of pinhole pupilloplasty. A clear, focused image is obtained when the rays from the central cornea are focused on the retina. (Reprinted with permission from Narang P, Agarwal A, Kumar DA, Agarwal A. Pinhole pupilloplasty: Small-aperture optics for higher-order corneal aberrations. *J Cataract Refract Surg*. 2019;45[5]:539-543. doi: 10.1016/j.jcrs.2018.12.007)

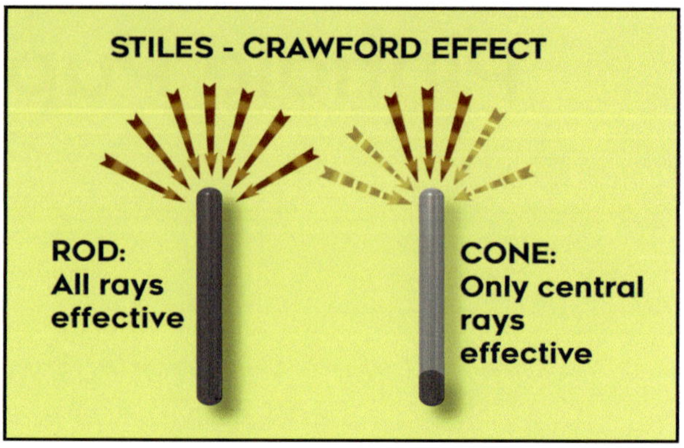

Figure 13-2. Stiles-Crawford effect.

Role of Purkinje Images in Pinhole Pupilloplasty

Theoretically, there are 4 Purkinje images (P1, P2, P3, and P4), but clinically, due to P1 and P2 overlapping each other, only 3 are appreciated (P1, P3, and P4). The P1 image is formed from the anterior surface of cornea and is right and upright. The P3 image is formed by the anterior surface of the lens or intraocular lens (IOL) and is large and upright. The P4 image is formed by the posterior surface of the lens/IOL and is inverted. In a pseudophakic eye, the P1 image should, ideally, be placed between the P3 and P4 images. A deviation from this, or proximity of the P1 image to either P3 or P4, indicates tilt or decentration of the IOL.

Purkinje Image From Light Reflex of Surgical Microscope

Intraoperatively, the surgical microscope projects the light reflex on the eye that translates into the formation of Purkinje images. As the Lumera microscope (Zeiss) projects 3 reflexes, each Purkinje image is a collection of 3 light reflexes. The main illumination light is in the top of the triad and the light from the 2 coaxial tubes form the 2 side reflexes.[4] The iris tissue is aimed to surround the P1 reflex with the help of pinhole pupilloplasty, thereby achieving a customized small pinhole pupil (Video 13-2).

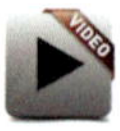

Surgical Technique of Achieving a Pinhole

The procedure of pinhole pupilloplasty can be performed with any technique—McCannel, Siepser, or cerclage—but the authors employ the single-pass four-throw technique (SFT)[5] for achieving a pinhole pupil (Figure 13-3 and Video 13-1).

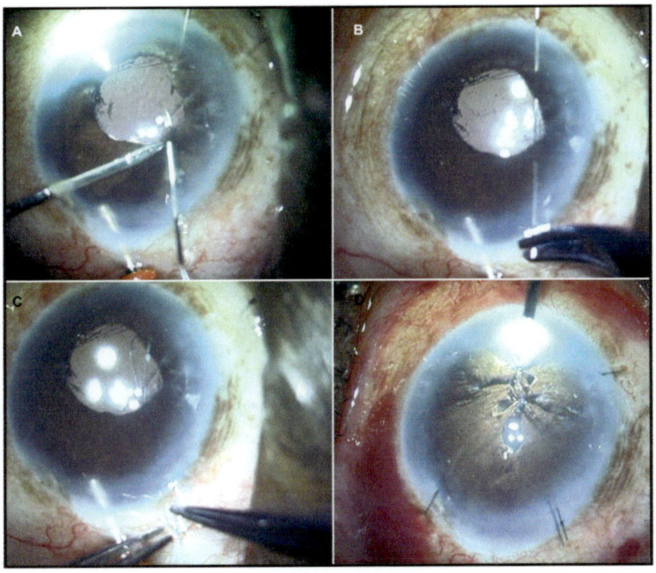

Figure 13-3. Clinical image demonstrating the SFT technique to achieve a pinhole pupil. (A) The proximal portion of the iris from where the 10-0 suture is to be passed is held with end-opening forceps. SFT is performed. The 10-0 needle engages the proximal iris tissue and a 26/30-gauge needle is introduced from the paracentesis in the opposite direction and engages the distal iris tissue. (B) The 10-0 needle is being pulled out of the eye. (C) The suture loop is withdrawn with a Sinskey hook and the suture end is passed through the loop 4 times. (D) A pinhole pupil that envelopes the P1 reflex in its center is achieved.

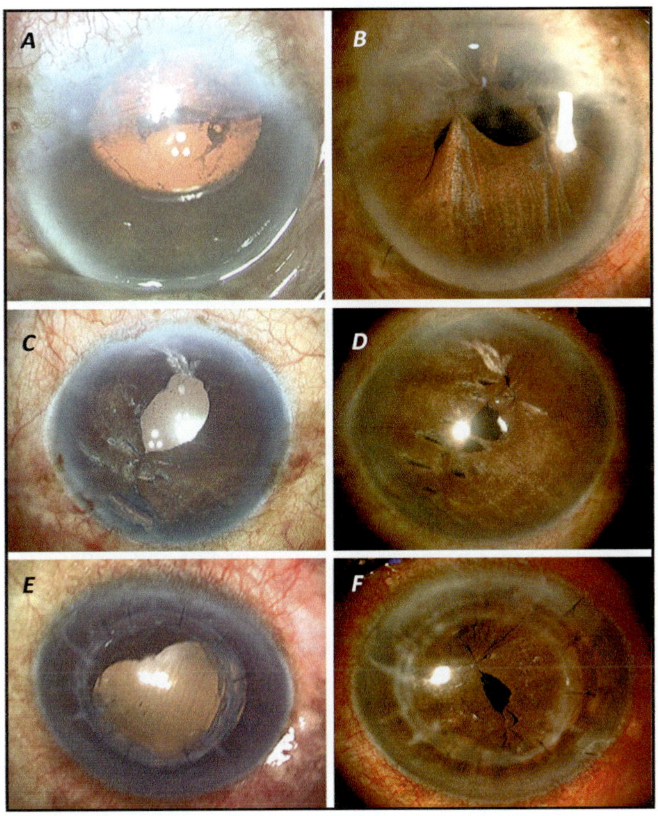

Figure 13-4. Pre- and postoperative images of cases that underwent pinhole pupilloplasty. (A) Preoperative image of a case with high irregular astigmatism following a patch graft. Pentacam (Oculus) showed astigmatism of 24.2 diopters (D). (B) Postoperative image of the case (as shown in A) with pinhole pupilloplasty. (C) Preoperative image of the case after glass intraocular foreign body removal. Pentacam shows astigmatism of 4.4 D. Patient had immense glare and decreased vision. (D) Postoperative image of the same case (shown in C) after pinhole pupilloplasty. Postoperative vision was 6/6 without glasses on Snellen chart. (E) Preoperative image of a case with high irregular astigmatism following a penetrating keratoplasty procedure. Pentacam demonstrated astigmatism of 26.6 D. (F) Postoperative image after phacoemulsification, IOL placement, and pinhole pupilloplasty (shown in E). (Reprinted with permission from Narang P, Agarwal A, Kumar DA, Agarwal A. Pinhole pupilloplasty: Small-aperture optics for higher-order corneal aberrations. *J Cataract Refract Surg*. 2019;45[5]:539-543. doi: 10.1016/j.jcrs.2018.12.007)

The multiple quadrant approach is necessary to achieve a pinhole pupil. The SFT procedure is performed and a minimum of 3 attempts or more are required to create a pinhole pupil. Often, the iris tissue overlaps the P1 reflex of Lumera microscope (Figure 13-4). Under these circumstances, a vitrectomy probe is used to reshape the pupil (see Video 13-2).

Pinhole Pupilloplasty and Chord Mu (µ)

With the procedure of pinhole pupilloplasty, the pupillary axis and visual axis are brought close to each other. Angle kappa is the angular distance formed between the pupillary axis and the visual axis. Recently, instead of using the terminology of angle kappa, a more appropriate term, called *chord mu,* has been suggested. Chord mu represents the chord length between the pupillary axis and the visual axis that has been found to decrease following pinhole pupilloplasty. Chord mu is specifically defined by Chang and Waring[4] as the chord distance between P1 and the center of the pupil when viewed through the cornea. The cornea magnifies and deviates the ray or the normal value as it appears through the cornea that is known, as an *apparent chord mu* is different from the *actual chord mu* that is measured at the iris plane.[6,7] The IOL Master (Zeiss) and LenStar (Haag-Streit) measure apparent chord mu as the mean value of 0.30 mm nasal and about 0.05 mm inferior, so the mean chord mu is 0.30 mm on the hypotenuse. The standard deviation is about 0.15, therefore 97.5% of the population is less than 0.60 mm. This is the value that is taken into consideration when halos and glare are experienced from a too large chord mu. On the other hand, the Pentacam uses Scheimpflug and gives the *actual distance* between the visual axis and the center of the pupil at the iris plane, which is about 0.20 mm with a standard deviation of 0.11, so the value for Scheimpflug is 0.42 mm (not 0.60 mm).

Calculation of Chord Mu (µ)

Pentacam denotes the X and Y coordinates of the pupil center in its analytic report. Chord mu is calculated as the square root of the sum of X and Y coordinates. The following formula is applicable: $C = \sqrt{(x^2 + y^2)}$. The resultant value C denotes the value of chord mu.

Discussion

The principle of pinhole has been applied to the cornea as well as to the placement of IOLs.[8-12] With pinhole pupilloplasty, the principle is applied to the pupil and iris (Figure 13-5). When pinhole pupilloplasty is performed, the coaxially sighted corneal light reflex axis and the line of sight converge at the fixation point. Therefore, chord mu decreases as the frame of reference moves anteriorly toward the observer and fixation point. In clinical practice, the change in chord mu between the lens–IOL plane (actual chord mu) and the corneal plane (apparent chord mu) is typically not significant. Apparent chord mu as seen through the cornea and actual chord mu as measured by Scheimpflug are different, just as the apparent and actual pupil size vary. The normal apparent chord mu as measured on the LenStar and IOL Master is 0.30 mm ± 0.15 mm. The actual chord mu as measured on the Pentacam or Galilei (Ziemer) is 0.20 mm ± 0.11 mm. When screening patients to avoid glare and halos with diffractive multifocal IOLs, the upper limit for apparent chord mu is 0.60 mm (mean +2 SD) and for actual chord mu is 0.42 mm (mean +2 SD). When pinhole pupilloplasty is performed, the distance between the pupillary axis and visual axis decreases (ie, the chord length decreases) and this indirectly translates into improved image and visual quality.

Studies have revealed a significant decrease in the horizontal and vertical pupil diameter, along with a significant change in the pre- and postoperative uncorrected visual acuity[1] and chord mu following pinhole pupilloplasty. When the patient is operated under peribulbar block, the subject-fixated coaxially sighted corneal light reflex, which is a more precise description of the coaxially sighted corneal light reflex concept, is not visualized. Rather, a coaxially sighted corneal light reflex is seen and pinhole pupilloplasty is performed taking that into consideration. An alternative to this could be that preoperative corneal marking is done along the pupillary center and pinhole pupilloplasty is then centered around it intraoperatively.

One should not make the pupil too small, otherwise diffraction will occur (Figure 13-6). The ideal pinhole size is about 1.5 mm.

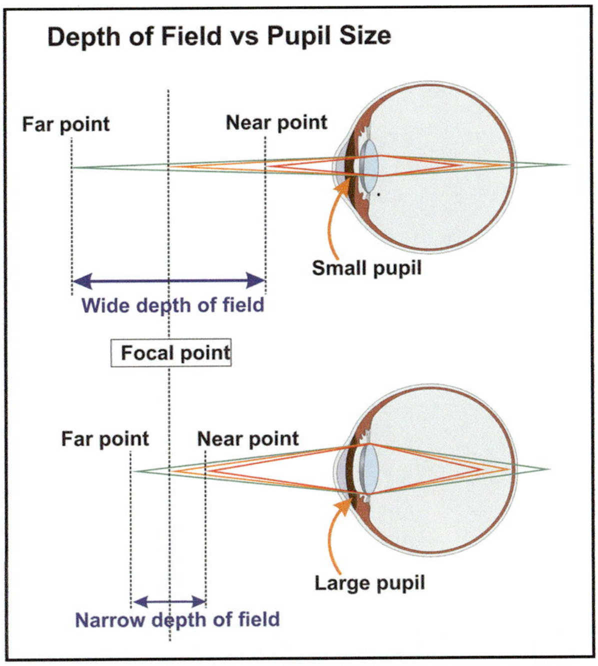

Figure 13-5. Pinhole pupil creates an extended depth of focus.

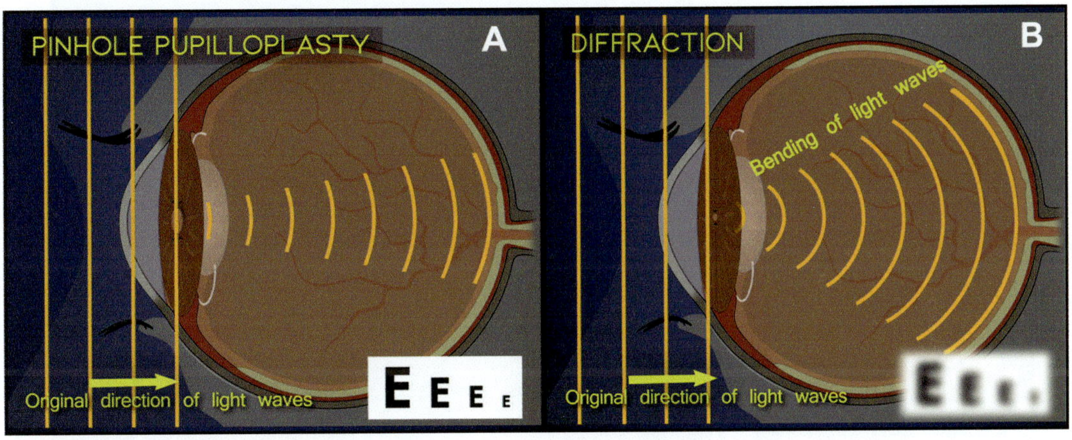

Figure 13-6. Diffraction will occur if the pinhole is too small. The ideal size is 1.5 mm.

The advantages of performing a pinhole pupilloplasty (Figure 13-7) is that no special device is needed to create the pinhole effect, the procedure is surgeon dependent, effective, and can be mastered easily (Figure 13-8). The immense improvement of visual quality in cases with higher order corneal aberrations following pinhole pupilloplasty makes it a pragmatic choice in optimizing vision for patients. One can also examine the fundus in patients after pinhole pupilloplasty (Figure 13-9), as the pupil dilates a little if performed using the SFT pupilloplasty technique.

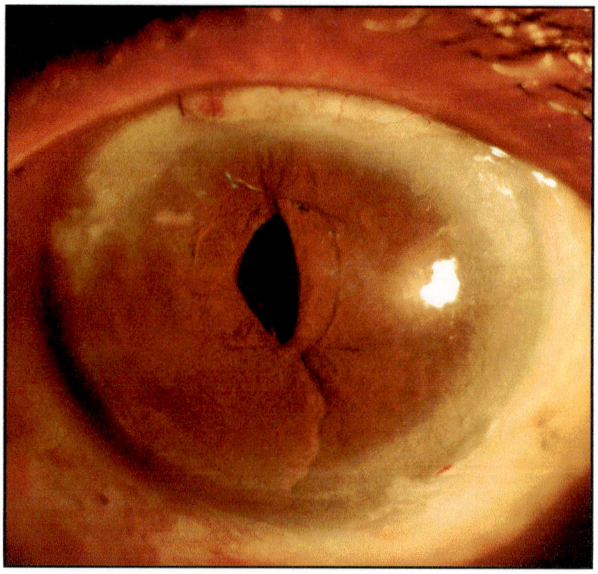

Figure 13-7. Case of pre-Descemet's endothelial keratoplasty with pinhole pupilloplasty. Vision was 20/20 and J1 without glasses because extended depth of focus was created.

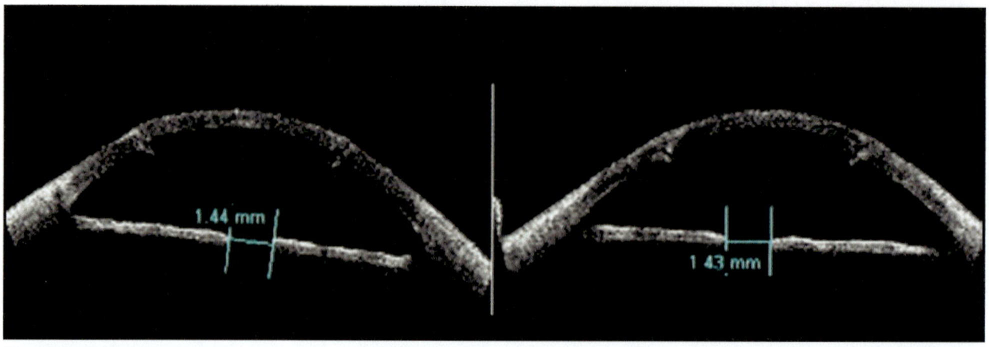

Figure 13-8. Anterior segment optical coherence tomography demonstrating the pinhole pupil created by pinhole pupilloplasty.

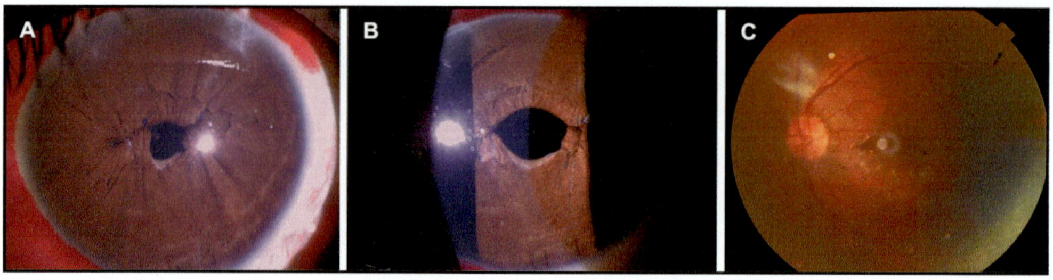

Figure 13-9. Pinhole pupilloplasty case before and after dilatation. (A) Pinhole pupilloplasty. (B) Same case after dilatation. Notice pupil dilates a bit if pinhole pupilloplasty is performed with the SFT pupilloplasty technique. (C) Fundus photo of patient following pinhole pupilloplasty.

Case Presentation

Pinhole Pupilloplasty in Keratoconus

Priya Narang, MS; Amar Agarwal, MS, FRCS, FRCOphth; and Ashvin Agarwal, MBBS, MS

A 40-year-old man presented with a history of keratoconus with an uncorrected visual acuity of counting fingers 1 m. The case was investigated and a detailed slit-lamp examination along with Pentacam assessment was performed. The patient had astigmatism of 5 D with an eccentric cone.

Pinhole pupilloplasty was performed for the case, along with lens removal and implantation of a foldable IOL. The pinhole pupilloplasty was centered on the P1 and the multiple quadrant approach was adopted (Figure 13-10). The postoperative visual acuity of the case was 6/12 on Snellen chart with N4 vision for near distance (Video 13-3).

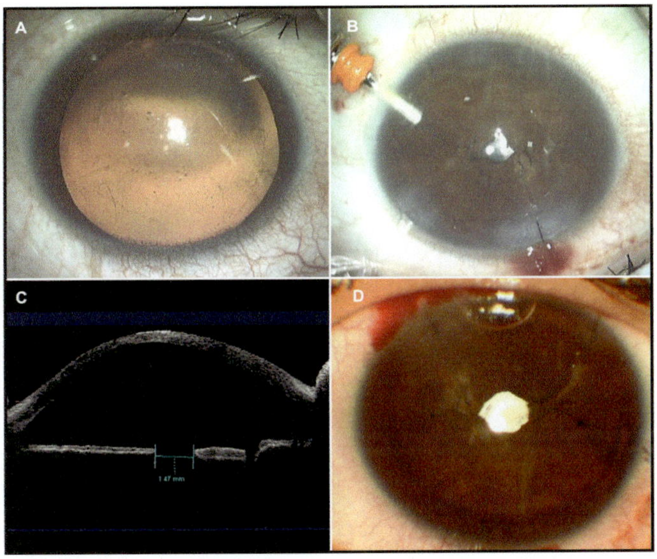

Figure 13-10. Clinical case of a young patient with keratoconus. (A) Case of keratoconus. Vision counting fingers 1 m without glasses. (B) Intraoperative centration of pupil on P1. (C) Anterior segment optical coherence tomography depicts the pupillary aperture of 1.47 mm in the postoperative period. (D) Postoperative day 2 image of the case. Vision is 6/12 N4 without glasses.

References

1. Narang P, Agarwal A, Kumar DA, Agarwal A. Pinhole pupilloplasty (PPP): small aperture optics for higher order corneal aberrations. *J Cataract Refract Surg.* 2019;45(5):539-543.
2. Westheimer, G. Directional sensitivity of the retina: 75 years of Stiles-Crawford effect. *Proc Biol Sci.* 2008;275(1653):2777-2786.
3. Stiles WS, Crawford BH. The luminous efficiency of rays entering the eye pupil at different points. *Proc R Soc Kind [Biol].* 1993;112(778):428-450.
4. Chang DH, Waring GO. The subject-fixated coaxially sighted corneal light reflex: a clinical marker for centration of refractive treatments and devices. *Am J Ophthalmol.* 2014;158(5):863-874.
5. Narang P, Agarwal A. Single-pass four-throw technique for pupilloplasty. *Eur J Ophthalmol.* 2017;27(4):506-508.
6. Holladay JT, Calogero D, Hilmantel G, et al. Special report: American Academy of Ophthalmology Task Force summary statement for measurement of tilt, decentration, and chord length. *Ophthalmology.* 2017;124(1):144-146.
7. Holladay JT, Simpson MJ. Negative dysphotopsia: causes and rationale for prevention and treatment. *J Cataract Refract Surg.* 2017;43:263-275.
8. Trindade CLC, Trindade LC. Novel pinhole intraocular implant for the treatment of irregular corneal astigmatism and severe light sensitivity after penetrating keratoplasty. *J Cataract Refract Surg.* 2015;3:4-7.
9. Trindade CC, Trindade BC, Trindade FC, Werner L, Osher R, Santhiago MR. New pinhole sulcus implant for the correction of irregular corneal astigmatism. *J Cataract Refract Surg.* 2017;43:1297-1306
10. Dick HB, Piovella M, Vukich J, Vilupuru S, Lin L, Clinical Investigators. Prospective multicenter trial of a small-aperture intraocular lens in cataract surgery. *J Cataract Refract Surg.* 2017;43:956-968
11. Schultz T, Dick HB. Small-aperture intraocular lens implantation in a patient with an irregular cornea. *J Refract Surg.* 2016;32:706-708.
12. Trindade BLC, Trindade FC, Trindade CLC, Santhiago MR. Phacoemulsification with intraocular pinhole implantation associated with Descemet membrane endothelial keratoplasty to treat failed full-thickness graft with dense cataract. *J Cataract Refract Surg.* 2018;44:1280-1283.

Please visit www.routledge.com/9781630917265 to access additional material.

14

Tools for Repair of the Iris

Brandon D. Ayres, MD

KEYWORDS

cerclage, diathermy for iris repair, iris repair, pupilloplasty, vitrectomy for iris repair

Iris damage is not an uncommon complication of intraocular surgery. Floppy iris syndrome, as well as instruments such as iris hooks, rings, phacoemulsification needles, and vitrectors, can cause intraoperative trauma to the iris. Blunt and penetrating ocular trauma can also cause severe trauma to the iris and other intraocular structures. In these cases, iris repair[1-5] can be challenging. Fortunately, with the right tools, material, and knowledge, it can also be quite rewarding for both the patient and doctor (Videos 14-1 and 14-2).

SUTURE MATERIAL

Having the right suture material and needle is critical to making iris repair a success. Generally, a 10-0 polypropylene suture is the preferred suture for iris repair. The needle is as important as the suture material. A variety of needles are available on a 10-0 polypropylene suture. Needle selection will depend on the technique used. An iridodialysis repair will mostly require the use of straight needles, while a pupilloplasty or cerclage will generally use long, curved needles (Figure 14-1). The design of the needle is also important to consider. A cutting needle may cause large holes to form in the iris tissue, thus making repair difficult. Taper-cut or spatulated needles are preferred as they minimize trauma to the iris tissue. Double-armed sutures are preferred when mattress sutures are being placed. These can easily be converted to single-armed needles by removing a needle (Figure 14-2).

Agarwal A, Agarwal A, eds. *Mastering Iris Repair: A Video Textbook of Iris Repair and Pupilloplasty Techniques* (pp 145-152).

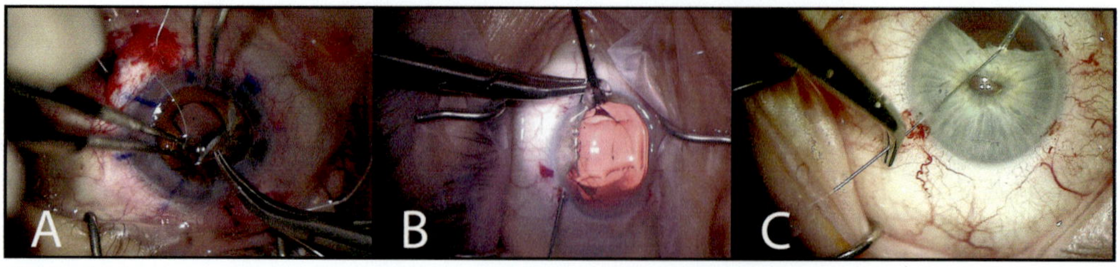

Figure 14-1. (A) A small vascular needle is used with a 10-0 polypropylene suture to perform an open-sky repair of the iris combined with corneal transplant. (B) A long, curved reverse cutting needle is used to help with an iris cerclage suture in a patient with an atonic iris. (C) Long, straight needles are docked into the 25-gauge guide needle to help with the repair of an iridodialysis.

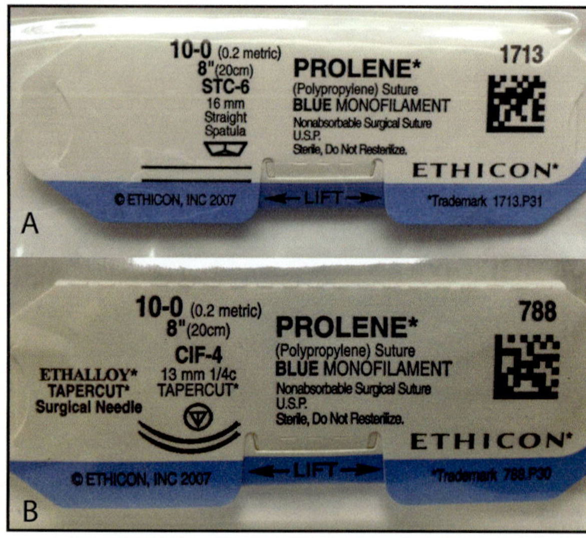

Figure 14-2. (A, B) Two commonly used 10-0 polypropylene sutures. The needle used will depend on the chosen technique of iris repair.

Suture Recovery Devices

Many techniques for iris repair require the use of a polypropylene suture. A multitude of different tying techniques have been described that allow knots to be tied in the anterior chamber. In the majority of cases, suture material will have to be recovered through a small incision and then tied in such a way to allow the knot to secure to an intraocular structure. This process is the basis of the McCannel suture technique, as well as the Siepser sliding knot. Suture recovery can be surprisingly difficult. Several tools have been designed to assist with this challenging and critical step of surgery.

Any surgical hook, such as a Sinskey or Kuglen, can be used to help snare suture material in the anterior chamber and recover it through a separate incision. At times, the hook will catch on the exit wound making it difficult to remove from the eye or the hook will release the suture in the anterior chamber. A variety of surgical instruments have been designed to help make suture recovery easier. A microhook, often called a *Bonn Micro Iris Hook* (Katena), is a small rounded hook that can be placed through a limbal incision. This hook is used to recover the suture from the anterior chamber and can be externalized through a limbal incision (Figure 14-3).

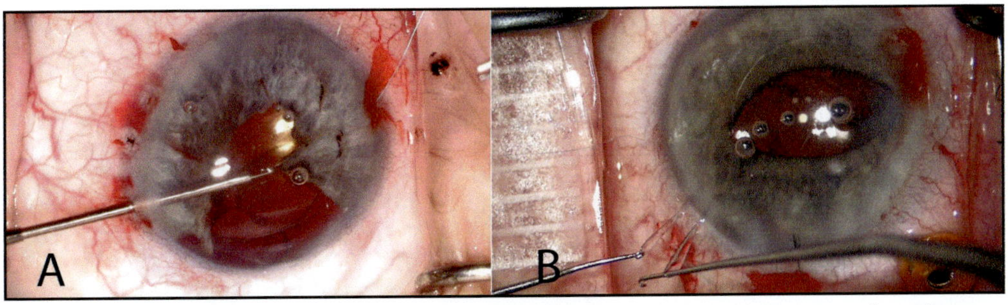

Figure 14-3. (A) An intraocular snare is used to recover a suture during an iridoplasty procedure. The snare is designed to allow the suture to slide preventing traction on the iris tissue and allow easy removal through a small incision. (B) A microhook is used to recover a 10-0 polypropylene suture from the anterior chamber. The small hooks allow the suture to be snared and removed through small limbal wounds. (Reprinted with permission from Nicole Fram, MD.)

Intraocular Forceps

It is essential to have a few specialized tools for successful iris repair. Ideally, microinstrumentation for anterior segment surgery will be able to fit through a small 1.0 to 1.5 mm incision (23 to 25 gauge). The instrument also needs to be sturdy enough to grab and manipulate tissue without bending. Many of the incisions for iris repair will be made at the limbus, so a gentle curve in the shaft of the instrument is helpful for surgeon ergonomics. The head of the instrument will determine its function. Iris tissue is fragile, so a typical toothed forceps design will cause trauma to the iris. Most forceps for use in iris repair will have a serrated jaw, a grasping finger, or a smooth finish to prevent trauma to the iris.

Depending on the surgical needs, microforceps can be very helpful with iris repair. The serrated forceps can be used to grasp the iris border with minimal trauma to tissue. Pupil border repair, cerclage sutures, and dialysis repair can all be assisted with a serrated microforceps. A microforceps with a downturned finger can also be helpful in iris repair. This microfinger-style forceps are very helpful in grasping iris stroma and pupil border and can be used with iridodialysis repair, cerclage, and other iris reconstructive procedures. In many cases, the decision to use a microfinger, smooth, or serrated forceps will be determined by the clinical situation and surgeon preference (Figure 14-4).

Microscissors

Microscissors are a critical tool in iris repair. Similar to microforceps, the scissors will need to be placed through small incisions. The blades of the scissors can be either straight or curved. Depending on the purpose of the scissors, the shaft may also be curved or straight. In many cases, the scissors are quite fragile and can only be used for cutting of tissue or fine suture in the eye. Cutting an IOL with microscissors will dull and bend the cutting blades rendering them useless for more delicate surgery.

Microscissors have numerous uses in iris repair. In many cases, they are necessary for cutting suture ends from intraocular knots. The ability to cut suture in the eye is essential, as it prevents the need to pull the knot to a limbal incision, which will cause tension and may damage iris tissue. In cases where the iris is incarcerated into a corneal wound (surgical or traumatic), the iris may need to be cut free. Microscissors are quite helpful in cutting the iris tissue free from the corneal wounds. After it is freed, the iris tissue can be reapproximated with sutures. In some cases of coloboma repair, the iris tissue will have to be cut before adequate repair can be performed (Figure 14-5).

Microscissors with curved blades can also be helpful in iris repair and reconstruction. The curved scissors can be used in place of a straight bladed scissor in many repair procedures, especially when reconstructing the pupil border. The curved blade assists in making a curved incision simplifying the reconstruction process (Figure 14-6).

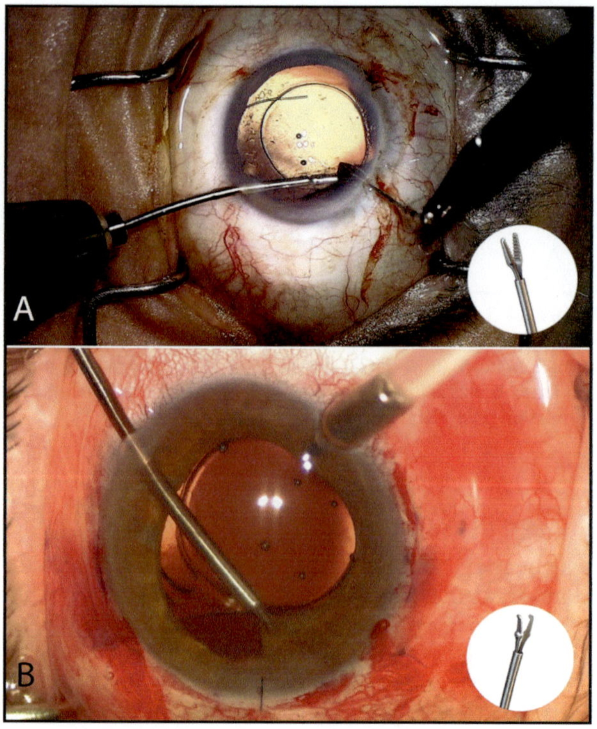

Figure 14-4. (A) A serrated microforceps is used to help grasp the iris during placement of a cerclage suture. The atraumatic forceps help grasp the iris without trauma. (B) Microforceps with a microfinger are used to help grasp the iris border. The downturned finger can be helpful in grasping the iris for repair. The curved shaft of the forceps allows for easier manipulation and placement in the anterior chamber. (Reprinted with permission from MST Surgical.)

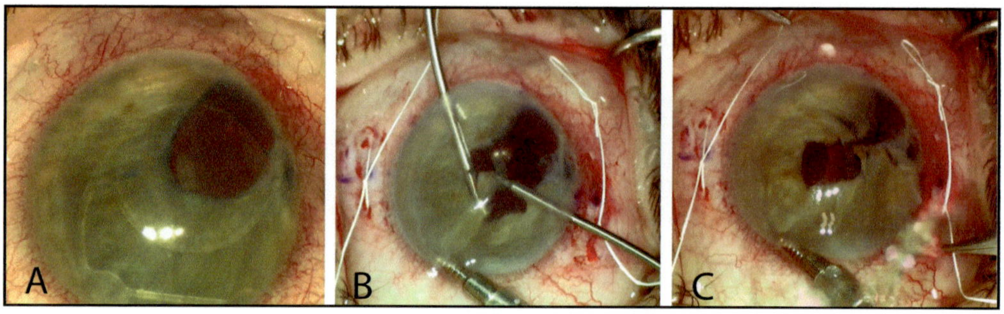

Figure 14-5. (A) A patient with an irregular pupil prior to repair. (B) Microscissors are used to make relaxing incisions in the iris stroma, creating a new pupil for the patient. (C) The postoperative appearance of the reconstructed pupil.

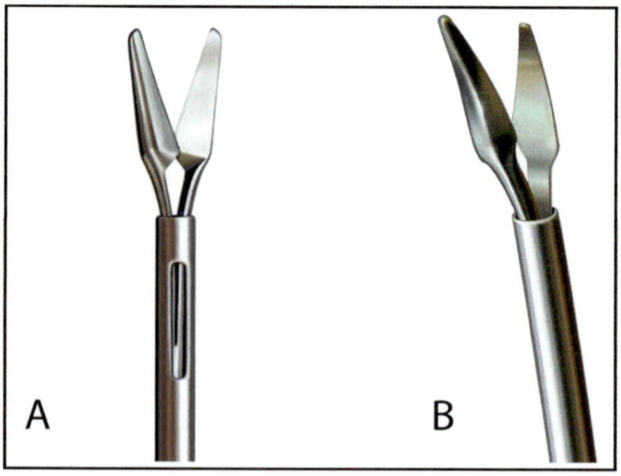

Figure 14-6. (A) Straight microscissors and (B) curved microscissors. Both instruments are valuable in iris repair surgery. (Reprinted with permission from MST Surgical.)

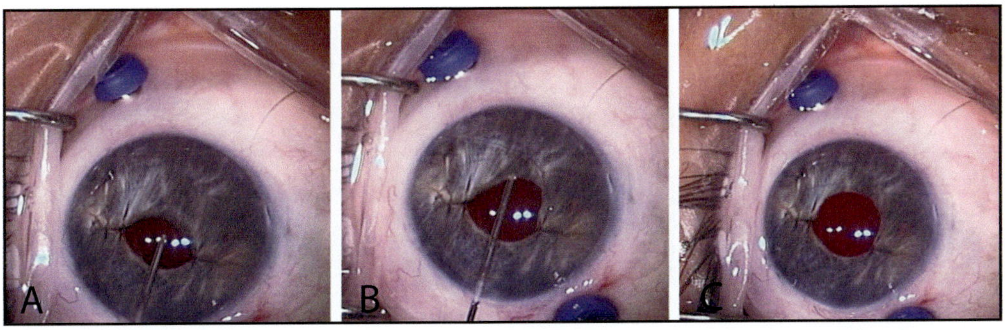

Figure 14-7. (A) A patient after suture repair of the iris left with an irregular shaped pupil. (B) The vitrector is used to carefully shape the iris border leaving (C) a round and well-centered pupil. (Reprinted with permission from Michael E. Snyder, MD.)

Iris Vitrectomy

In most cases, iris reconstruction relies on reapproximation and reshaping of the iris to re-establish the iris diaphragm; sometimes, it is necessary to remove iris tissue. The anterior vitrector can be a valuable tool in selectively removing iris tissue to create or center the pupil. A 23-, 25-, or 27-gauge vitrector can be used for iris tissue removal. Use a high cut rate and low aspiration rate with the vitrector for excellent control and to ensure that not too much iris is pulled. Any time the vitrector is used for iris tissue removal, it is helpful to have an infusion line in the anterior chamber or in the pars plana (Figure 14-7).

Intraocular Diathermy

Traditionally, cautery is used during ophthalmic surgery for hemostasis. Another use of the intraocular diathermy is in iris reconstruction. Using low levels of cautery on the iris stroma will cause the iris fibrils to shrink. Strategically cauterizing the iris stroma can be performed to help round, reshape, and pull the pupil. This technique is very similar to using the argon laser to heat and shape the pupil but can be done in the operating room. Iris cautery is often used to augment suture repairs where the pupil is left slightly peaked or decentered (Figure 14-8). The shaping effect on the iris stroma is long lasting, but will cause small areas of pigment loss. These spots from iris cautery can be visible, especially in light-colored irises, but rarely cause symptomatic glare.

Ophthalmic Viscosurgical Device

Ophthalmic viscosurgical devices (OVDs) are used in most anterior segment surgical procedures to act as a space filling material and protect the corneal endothelium. OVD in iris repair serves the same function with one useful additional feature—the cannula can be used to help recover the needle from the 10-0 polypropylene suture. In cases where the needle on the polypropylene suture is exiting the anterior chamber through a paracentesis, it is very easy to mistakenly catch a fibril of the corneal stroma. This inadvertent incarceration of tissue makes tying a sliding knot or continuation of a cerclage suture very difficult. Placing the cannula through the exit wound and docking the needle into the lumen of the cannula will allow the needle to exit the eye without fear of catching the cornea on the way out. In this way, the OVD itself is a tool for maintenance of the anterior chamber, and the cannula a surgical tool for suture recovery (Figure 14-9).

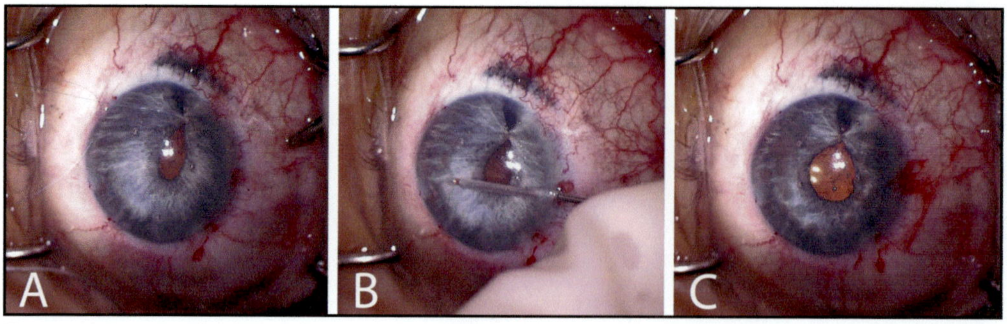

Figure 14-8. (A) A suture iris repair following traumatic injury. The sutures leave the iris severely peaked and decentered. (B) Intraocular diathermy is used to reshape and round the pupil border. (C) The iris suture repair is augmented by intraocular diathermy. Note the spots of depigmentation caused by the tip of the cautery device.

Figure 14-9. During placement of a cerclage suture, the OVD is used to help maintain the anterior chamber, and the cannula is used to help guide the needle out of the paracentesis. This technique prevents the needle from grabbing cornea fibers as it exits the eye.

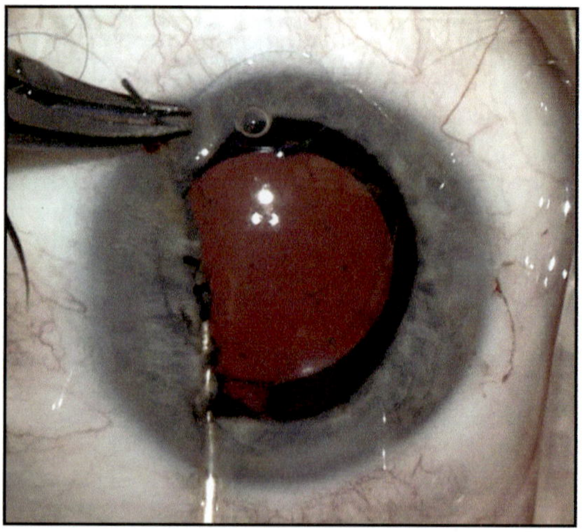

Conclusion

Iris repair is much more an art than a science. It is essential to have a firm understanding of what tools and techniques are available and how to use them. Armed with the proper surgical tools, surgical training, and creative vision, surgeons will find iris repair enjoyable and rewarding.

Case Presentation

Vitrector Used to Create a Pinhole Pupil for Refractive Surprise

Priya Narang, MS; Ashvin Agarwal, MBBS, MS; and Amar Agarwal, MS, FRCS, FRCOphth

A 52-year-old woman had cataract surgery and subsequently developed a refractive surprise. Twenty years back the patient had LASIK done. Preoperative vision was uncorrected visual acuity (UCVA): 6/60; best corrected visual acuity: +2.00; sphere: 6/18. Cataract surgery was performed with phaco. A +24 diopters intraocular lens (IOL) was implanted after biometry using the ASCRS calculator.

At 3 months postoperatively, the patient's UCVA was 6/24 with +2.00 -2.5 @ 75 degrees patient improved to 6/9 (Figure 14-10A). Pentacam (Oculus) photo shows a well-centered ablation after LASIK. The patient was unhappy with her vision.

Instead of exchanging the IOL, we performed a pinhole pupilloplasty to solve the refractive surprise. Her vision improved from 6/24 to 6/9 without glasses (Figure 14-10B). The patient had N6 for near vision due to the extended depth of focus of the pinhole pupilloplasty (Video 14-3).

In cases of refractive surprise, patients do well with pinhole pupilloplasty if their main issue is astigmatism. The vitrector helps to make the Purkinje image P1 match the pupillary center.

If the patient has only a refractive component, then the results will not be as great and vision will improve from CF to 6/60. In those cases, we prefer to do an IOL exchange.

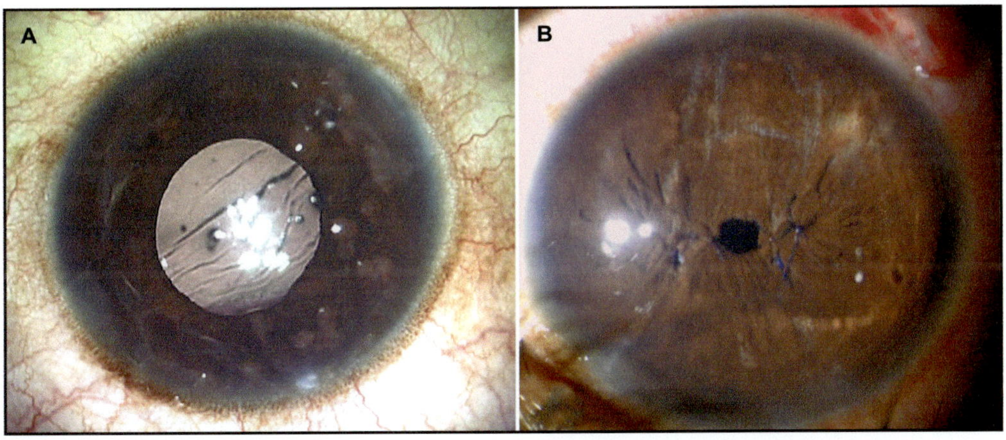

Figure 14-10. Pinhole pupilloplasty for refractive surprise. (A) Case of phaco surgery performed in an eye that had LASIK 20 years prior. The patient experienced a refractive surprise. Refraction was UCVA 6/24 and with +2.00 - 2.5 @ 75 degrees, best corrected visual acuity was 6/9. (B) Postoperative day 3. UCVA was 6/9 N6 after pinhole pupilloplasty. The vitrector probe was used to see that the Purkinje image P1 of the microscope matched the pupillary center.

References

1. Nunziata BR. Repair of iridodialysis using a 17-millimeter straight needle. *Ophthalmic Surg.* 1993;24(9):627-629.
2. Ogawa GS. The iris cerclage suture for permanent mydriasis: a running suture technique. *Ophthalmic Surg Lasers Imaging.* 1998;29(12):1001-1009.
3. Siepser SB. The closed chamber slipping suture technique for iris repair. *Ann Ophthalmol.* 1994;26:71-72.
4. Osher RH, Snyder ME, Cionni RJ. Modification of the Siepser slip-knot technique. *J Cataract Refract Surg.* 2005;31(6):1098-1100.
5. Narang P, Agarwal A. Single-pass four-throw technique for pupilloplasty. *Eur J Ophthalmol.* 2017;27(4):506-508.

Please visit www.routledge.com/9781630917265

to access additional material.

15

Pinhole Intraocular Lenses
All You Need to Know

Claudio Trindade, MD, PhD

Keywords

IC-8 IOL, pinhole intraocular lens, pinhole optics, pinhole, small aperture, small aperture intraocular lens, XtraFocus implant

Small aperture optics has become increasingly popular over the last decade. The first attempt to incorporate a pinhole mask into an intraocular lens (IOL) implant dates back to 1964, when renowned British ophthalmologist Peter Choyce revealed the Mark V implant (Rayner), an anterior chamber polymethyl methacrylate IOL with an embedded pinhole mask.[1] Four decades later, the Kamra pinhole corneal inlay (AcuFocus; Figure 15-1) was approved by the US Food and Drug Administration to treat presbyopia.[2] However, the intrastromal space did not seem to be the best physiological site for a pinhole mask, and a trend towards a posterior chamber pinhole IOL was observed. In 2014, the proof of concept of the XtraFocus pinhole implant (Morcher GmbH) was published[3] and AcuFocus presented the IC-8 pinhole IOL.[4] The purpose of this chapter is to highlight the technical details and indications of this new class of intraocular implants.

Background

The camera obscura, or dark chamber, is the starting point for all practical applications of the pinhole effect. First descriptions date back to 500 BCE, when Chinese philosopher Mo Ti described that the image of an object can be projected into a collecting surface of a dark room by entering a small opening in an opaque obstacle. The eye is a much more complex optical system. Its diaphragm, the iris, has an important role in not only controlling the light entrance but also

Agarwal A, Agarwal A, eds. *Mastering Iris Repair: A Video Textbook of Iris Repair and Pupilloplasty Techniques* (pp 153-160).

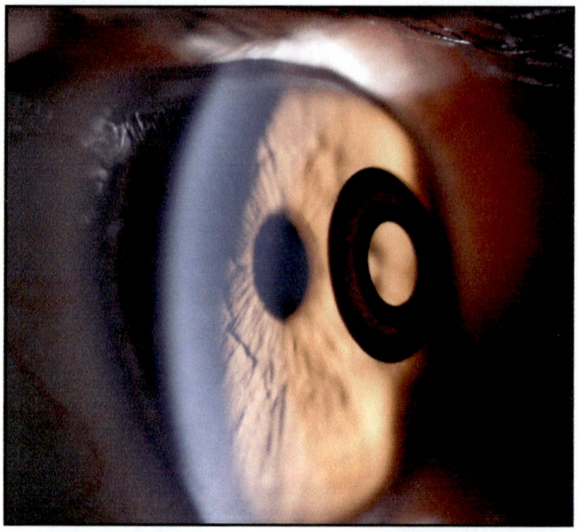

Figure 15-1. Kamra corneal inlay.

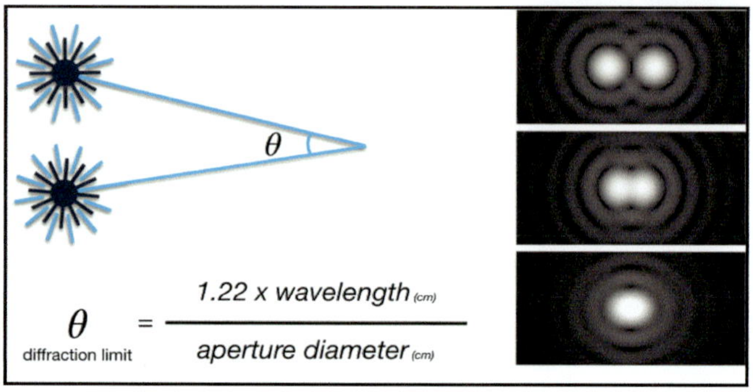

Figure 15-2. The diffraction limit of the eye is related to pupil size.

impacting the overall sharpness of the image formation. One important concept when dealing with iris aperture is *diffraction limit*. This term refers to the minimum angular separation between 2 light sources necessary for a perfect optical instrument to distinguish them individually. The accepted criterion for determining the diffraction limit to resolution based on this angle was developed by Lord Rayleigh in the 19th century. It is called the *Rayleigh criterion* (Figure 15-2). As noticed in the formula, the larger the aperture, the greater the ability to distinguish 2 adjacent light sources. This is one of the reasons why high-end telescopes have larger apertures. However, under imperfect optical conditions, like those frequently observed in the human eye, the angle of resolution is limited by the optical aberrations before diffraction starts playing a role. This is an important principle to keep in mind during patient selection for any small aperture IOL procedure. In 1991, Holladay et al studied the Snellen visual acuity as a function of pupil size and defocus.[5] Data analysis of more than 10,000 normal subjects revealed that patients with pupils as small as 1.0 mm could still reach 20/20 visual acuity while maintaining a very extended depth of focus. Another important consideration when dealing with pupil diameter is the difference between the apparent diameter and the actual diameter. Due to the magnification effect of the cornea, the apparent pupil diameter (as seen by the examiner) is approximately 14% larger than the actual pupil diameter.

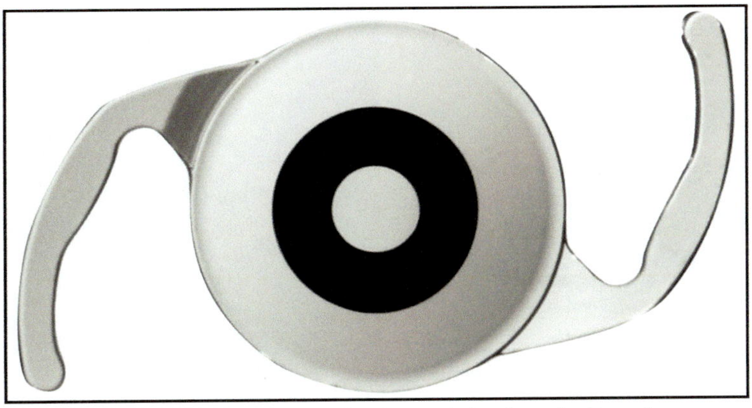

Figure 15-3. The IC-8 IOL. (Reprinted with permission from AcuFocus.)

Small Aperture Intraocular Lenses

Currently there are 2 models of small aperture IOLs commercially available.

IC-8 Intraocular Lens

The IC-8 IOL (Figure 15-3) is a single piece, hydrophobic acrylic IOL, with an optic size of 6 mm and an overall diameter of 12.5 mm, designed to be implanted in the capsular bag. The aspheric optic (negative spherical aberration of 0.27 mm) has an index of refraction of 1.48 and presents a 360-degree square edge. The haptics have a modified-C shape and are angulated 5 degrees. The pinhole mask, made of polyvinylidene difluoride and nanoparticles of carbon, is embedded into the acrylic matrix. The mask has an overall diameter of 3.23 mm with a central aperture of 1.36 mm. To avoid damage during the folding/unfolding process, the mask has 3200 microperforations, and an incision size of 3.5 mm is advisable. The IOL comes in +10.0 diopters (D) to +30.0 D. A toric version is not available. The IC-8 IOL, which received CE mark certification in 2014, is currently commercially available in Europe, Australia, and New Zealand.

XtraFocus Implant

The XtraFocus implant (Figure 15-4) is a single-piece implant made of a foldable black hydrophobic acrylic with an occlusive portion of 6 mm with a 1.3 mm central opening with no refractive power. It was designed to be implanted in the ciliary sulcus of pseudophakic eyes in a piggyback configuration. It can be used in combination with any IOL of choice, which must be placed inside the capsular bag. The device has specific characteristics for safe sulcus implantation, such as a larger overall diameter of 14.0 mm, rounded edges on the occlusive body, thin haptics (250 μm) with a polished and rounded profile, and an angulation of 16 degrees. The black acrylic is made of a combination of reactive dyes, which have functional groups that are covalently bonded to the polymeric acrylic structure. This black material has the unique feature of being transparent to infrared light, allowing examination of structures located behind the implant when using infrared-based equipment. The occlusive body has a very slim profile (180 μm around the pinhole) with a concave-convex shape to avoid contact with the primary IOL. Because of the reduced thickness, the device can be implanted through a 2.0 mm corneal incision. This implant, which received CE mark certification in 2016, is commercially available in Europe, Australia, New Zealand, and some countries in Latin America and the Middle East.

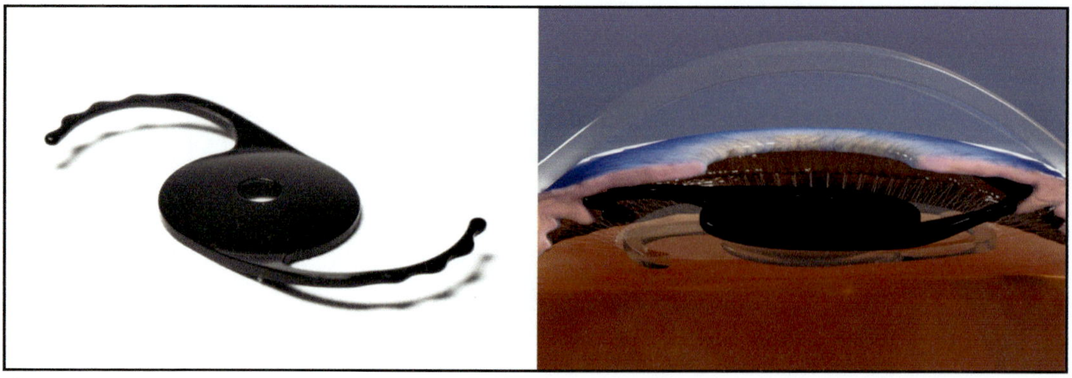

Figure 15-4. The XtraFocus pinhole implant.

Indications

Due to the ubiquitous nature of presbyopia, its treatment has always been the holy grail of the ophthalmic industry. It is well recognized that the depth of focus of the eye increases as pupil diameter decreases, and most studies with the IC-8 IOL focused on this application.[4,6] When the IC-8 is implanted monocularly in the nondominant eye in patients with an ideal refractive target of -0.75 D, a high level of spectacle independence and patient satisfaction has been observed. This allows for a continuous range of functional vision, with 79% of patients achieving 20/32 or better uncorrected near visual acuity, while still maintaining good uncorrected distance visual acuity.[6] Additionally, the pinhole effect can be very effective for the treatment of more challenging and complex cases of irregular corneal astigmatism. In 2017, the film *Tiny Hero Against the Evil Axis* (Video 15-1) won the American Society of Cataract and Refractive Surgery Film Festival Grand Prize with a case series in which the XtraFocus implant was used for the treatment of highly aberrated corneas.[7]

Postoperative radial keratotomy, penetrating keratoplasty, and patients who underwent LASIK, as well as those with ectasia and keratoconus, can benefit from this approach (Figure 15-5), especially those with a larger pupil diameter. Under those circumstances, a refractive target of -2.00 D is advisable. Although the pinhole effect neutralizes some astigmatism, postoperative penetrating keratoplasty and keratoconus patients with high astigmatism will benefit from a combination of a high-cylinder toric IOL with the XtraFocus implant. A confirmation of topographic stability is mandatory before surgery. It is important to highlight that in some cases of irregular astigmatism, conventional cataract surgery with a monofocal or toric IOL may give surprisingly good results. In those cases, the possibility of a secondary implantation is an important advantage of the XtraFocus implant.

The clinical benefit of pinhole IOLs in cases of irregular corneas is limited by the amount of high-order aberration. Patients with severe topographic irregularity and/or central corneal opacities may not achieve sufficient improvement in visual acuity with this treatment. In those cases, other corneal treatments, including a corneal graft, may be necessary.

Small aperture IOLs can also be used for the treatment of iris defects. Figure 15-6 shows a case of penetrating ocular injury with iris loss in which the XtraFocus implant was used. A reduction of glare, ghost images, and light sensitivity can be expected from this approach. Another interesting application of the XtraFocus implant is for the treatment of debilitating dysphotopsia after multifocal IOL implantation (Figure 15-7). Here, the piggyback design of the XtraFocus allows for a versatile solution in those cases where an IOL exchange presents significant risks (eg, previous posterior capsulotomy). This simple approach may be able to mitigate the symptoms, while preserving an extended range of functional vision (see Figure 15-7).

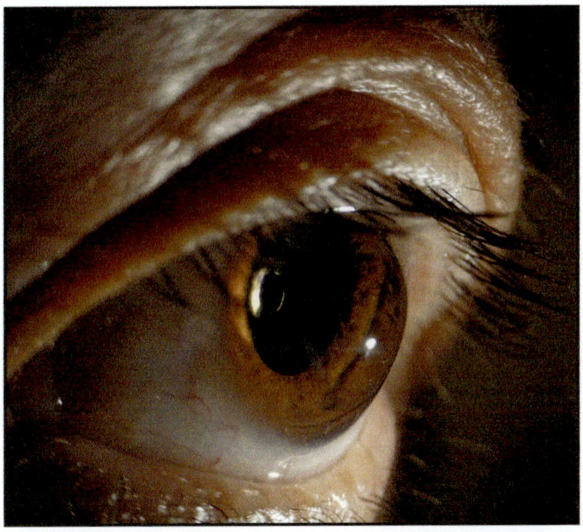

Figure 15-5. The XtraFocus implant inside an eye with keratoconus.

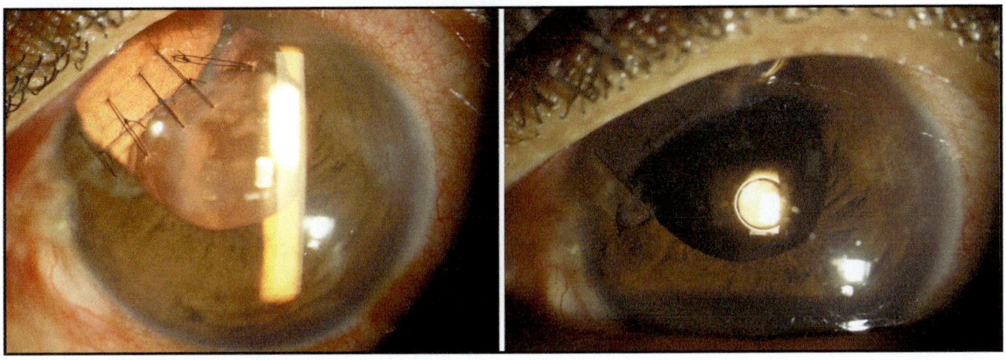

Figure 15-6. Pinhole IOLs can be used to correct iris defects.

Visual Field

Both models presented are implanted in close relation to the iris plane. This proximity to the natural diaphragm of the eye ensures minimal impact on the visual field. A reduction of overall retinal sensitivity, of approximately 2 decibels is expected after implantation.[6,8] As long as proper centration is achieved, no perception of visual field constriction is expected to occur after implantation of small aperture IOLs (Figure 15-8); however, the restriction of light entrance imposed by any small aperture intraocular implant may cause a sensation of darkening, especially under low-light conditions. The intensity of this symptom is widely variable, with multiple factors involved. An interesting paper from Artal and Manzanera[9] concluded that the reduction of brightness perception after a pinhole IOL implantation was less pronounced than what was expected based on the pupillary area.

Conclusion

Although the follow-up data is limited, the IOLs discussed in this chapter seem to be a very promising new class of intraocular implants. Clinical applications are numerous, including complex anterior segment conditions. Future studies will provide additional information, allowing for continuous improvement

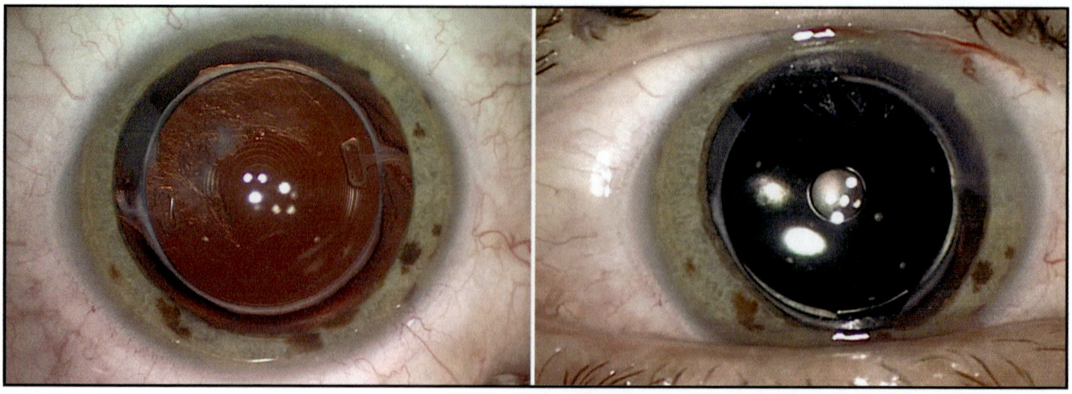

Figure 15-7. Extending the applications of pinhole optics: The XtraFocus Implant can be used to reduce dysphotopsia after multifocal IOL implantation.

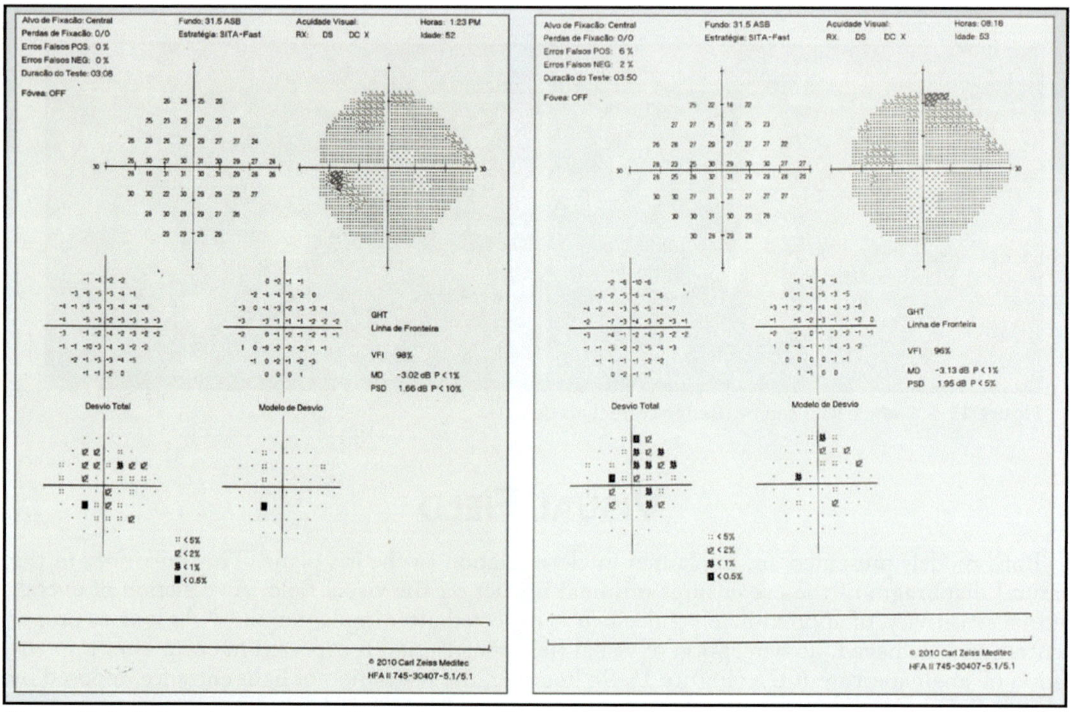

Figure 15-8. Slight reduction in overall retinal sensitivity with no clinical relevance.

Case Presentation

XtraFocus Intraocular Lens in a Postoperative Radial Keratotomy Eye

Priya Narang, MS; Ashvin Agarwal, MBBS, MS; and Amar Agarwal, MS, FRCS, FRCOphth

A 53-year-old male presented with a history of glare and a feeling of awkwardness while visualizing any object or a light source. Upon examination, the marks of radial keratotomy were seen on the cornea. The patient had also undergone cataract surgery recently with the placement of a foldable IOL into the capsular bag (Figure 15-9A).

The plan was to implant an XtraFocus IOL (Figure 15-9B) into the sulcus to overcome the aberrations arising from the corneal surface. The XtraFocus IOL acts like a pinhole that bars all the light rays arising from the peripheral corneal surface and helps to focus the central and paracentral rays (Figures 15-9C and 15-9D). Postoperatively, the patient was relieved of all the visual symptoms with subjective and objective improvement of visual image (Video 15-2).

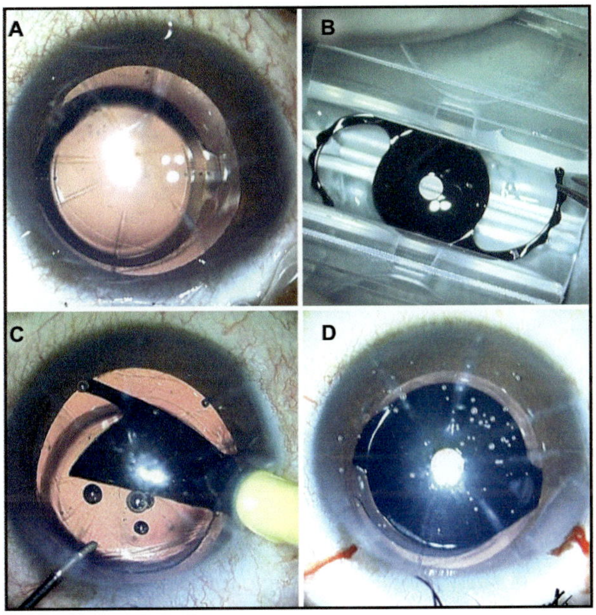

Figure 15-9. Trindade XtraFocus IOL in a postoperative radial keratotomy eye. (A) A case with 8 radial keratotomy marks with a foldable IOL placed in the capsular bag. (B) The XtraFocus IOL being loaded into the cartridge. (C) The XtraFocus IOL is injected into the sulcus. (D) The XtraFocus IOL is well placed into the sulcus and acts like a pinhole.

References

1. Choyce P. *Intra-ocular Lenses and Implants*. London, United Kingdom: H.K. Lewis;1964:211.
2. Dexl AK, Seyeddain O, Riha W, Hohensinn M, Hitzl W, Grabner G. Reading performance after implantation of a small-aperture corneal inlay for the surgical correction of presbyopia: two-year follow-up. *J Cataract Refract Surg*. 2011;37(3):525-531.
3. Trindade CLC, Trindade BLC. Novel pinhole intraocular implant for the treatment of irregular corneal astigmatism and severe light sensitivity after penetrating keratoplasty. *JCRS Online Case Reports*. 2015;3(1):4-7.
4. Grabner G, Ang RE, Vilupuru S. The small-aperture IC-8 intraocular lens: a new concept for added depth of focus in cataract patients. *Am J Ophthalmol*. 2015;160(6):1176-1184.
5. Holladay JT, Lynn MJ, Waring GO III, Gemmill M, Keehn GC, Fielding B. The relationship of visual acuity, refractive error, and pupil size after radial keratotomy. *Arch Ophthalmol*. 1991;109(1):70-76.
6. Dick HB, Piovella M, Vukich J, Vilupuru S, Lin L, Clinical I. Prospective multicenter trial of a small-aperture intraocular lens in cataract surgery. *J Cataract Refract Surg*. 2017;43(7):956-968.
7. Trindade CC, Trindade BC, Trindade FC, Werner L, Osher R, Santhiago MR. New pinhole sulcus implant for the correction of irregular corneal astigmatism. *J Cataract Refract Surg*. 2017;43(10):1297-1306.
8. Seyeddain O, Hohensinn M, Riha W, et al. Small-aperture corneal inlay for the correction of presbyopia: 3-year follow-up. *J Cataract Refract Surg*. 2012;38(1):35-45.
9. Artal P, Manzanera S. Perceived brightness with small apertures. *J Cataract Refract Surg*. 2018;44(6):734-737.

Please visit www.routledge.com/9781630917265

to access additional material.

16

Iris Tumors and Cysts

Sonal S. Chaugule, MS; Paul T. Finger, MD;
Santosh G. Honavar, MD, FACS, FRCOphth;
Dhivya Ashok Kumar, MD, FRCS, FICO, FAICO; and Athiya Agarwal, MD, DO

Keywords

cystotomy, cystectomy, iris cysts

Iris Tumors

Thought to be relatively uncommon, anteriorly located iris tumors are easily recognized by slit-lamp examination (Video 16-1). However, benign iridociliary cysts form the majority of acquired anterior segment tumors.[1] Iris melanomas are the most common primary anterior segment malignancy followed by ciliary body tumors with iris invasion. Iris melanomas are found in all races, but incidence is higher in White patients and those with lightly pigmented iris. Iris tumors can be broadly classified as cystic and solid (Box 16-1). This differentiation is evident on routine slit-lamp examination and gonioscopy as well as confirmed by high-frequency ultrasound biomicroscopy (UBM) and/or anterior segment optical coherence tomography (AS-OCT).

Diagnostic Features

Clinical Evaluation

Clinical evaluation for iris tumors involves a complete ophthalmic examination including, but not limited to, past medical history, best corrected visual acuity, tonometry, slit-lamp biomicroscopy, gonioscopy, ophthalmoscopy, and transillumination. A slit-lamp–assisted, high-resolution photograph and a detailed drawing of the tumor should be performed to document visible characteristics.[1] An iris tumor is described morphologically stating the shape (plateau,

Agarwal A, Agarwal A, eds. *Mastering Iris Repair: A Video Textbook of Iris Repair and Pupilloplasty Techniques* (pp 161-173).

Box 16-1. Classification of Iris Tumors

CYSTIC	SOLID
• Primary cystic lesions • Secondary cystic lesions	• Melanocytic ◦ Benign ◦ Malignant • Nonmelanocytic ◦ Benign ◦ Malignant • Miscellaneous

dome, mushroom), surface (smooth, rough, lobulated), color (white, yellow, orange, brown, black) dimensions (in millimeters), anatomic location or number of clock hours involved (superior, nasal, inferior, temporal), anteroposterior location (collarette, pupillary margin, mid-iris, and/or iris root), as well as involvement of adjacent structures (invasion of anterior chamber angle, and/or iris root, ciliary body involvement). Associated features include sector cataract, uveitis, dislocated lens, scleral invasion, extrascleral extension, and posterior involvement of the choroid.[1]

Ancillary Examination

The diagnosis of iris tumors has been greatly enhanced by advanced imaging techniques, such as high-frequency UBM[2-6] and AS-OCT,[7-9] as well as biopsy.[1,10,11]

Ultrasound Biomicroscopy

UBM is a high-frequency ultrasonographic imaging at frequency range of 20 to 50 MHz. UBM typically provides image resolution of approximately 25 μm and a depth penetration of 5 to 6 mm. This technique provides clinicians with high-resolution ultrasound images of the iris tumor surface, deep margins, and internal reflectivity. It also allows for quantitative evaluation of tumor dimensions, viewing of interstitial tumor borders, and, thus, evaluation of invasion/involvement of adjacent structures. [1,7-9,12-15]

Anterior Segment Optical Coherence Tomography

AS-OCT is a noncontact device that employs a superluminescent diode at 1310 nm wavelength for optical imaging with image resolution of 18 μm and a depth penetration of 3 to 4 mm.[7-9] It is a more comfortable imaging modality than UBM,[16] and a useful tool for evaluation of superficial, nonpigmented anterior surface tumors.[7] However, the diode-light cannot penetrate pigmented tissue, causing posterior shadowing and limited penetration.

Fluorescein Angiography

Iris fluorescein angiography can be a useful aid in the diagnosis of iris tumors.[17-20] The vascular pattern of the tumor can be compared to the normal vascular pattern of the surrounding and contralateral iris. The tumor's vascular network can be observed to leak into the aqueous when the tumor is hyperfluorescent. If fluorescein leakage is noted at the site, remote from the tumor, occult or multifocal tumors are suspected.[1] A disorganized vasculature exhibiting gross leakage of dye is suggestive of malignancy.[19,21]

Computed Tomography and Magnetic Resonance Imaging

Computed tomography and magnetic resonance imaging (MRI) can be helpful for delineation of scleral involvement and extrascleral extension of iris or iridociliary tumors.[22,23] They can be used to differentiate between solid tumors and certain benign conditions, such as foreign bodies, massive hemorrhage, and cystic lesions.[23-25]

Tumor Biopsy

Biopsy techniques for iris tumors include standard iridectomy, iridocyclectomy, fine-needle aspiration, and aspiration cutter–assisted transcorneal biopsy (Finger Iridectomy Technique).[1,11] The common indications for biopsy are atypical tumor, metastatic tumor with undetected primary tumor, and pathology diagnosis or genetic tumor analysis requested by the patient.[1,11,26]

Classification of Iris Tumors

Cystic Lesions

Primary iris cysts include neuroepithelial, pigment epithelial (IPE) cysts and stromal cysts.[27]

- Neuroepithelial cysts are the most common. Typically found at the junction of the iris root and ciliary body.[1,4] Rarely observed after maximal pupillary dilation using oblique slit-lamp biomicroscopy, these small, round, lucent cysts have thin, semi-transparent walls that can be seen to rest against the anterior lens capsule. The anterior margin of the neuroepithelial cyst can displace the overlying iris stroma, causing focal angle closure. However, there have been no reports of secondary angle-closure glaucoma (ACG). It has been our experience that neuroepithelial cysts can be multiple and bilateral. They can enlarge, stay the same size, or diminish. Though they can grow, no one has associated their growth with the development of malignancy; however, cysts have been noted anterior to ciliary body melanomas.[16]
- Primary IPE cysts, sometimes referred to as *iris pigment epithelial schisis*, arise from the posterior lamellae of the iris. They are pigmented and may be confused with ciliary body melanoma; however, the surface is smooth, avascular, and typically conformal to the lens and iris. IPE cysts can be categorized as pupillary margin, mid-zonal, peripheral, dislodged, and free floating.[28] Unlike, neuroepithelial iris cysts, their large size and broad contact with the iris stroma can cause angle closure with secondary glaucoma.[29,30]
    - Typically after pupillary dilation, IPE cysts can easily be visualized at the pupillary margin. Peripheral IPE cysts are typically hidden at the iridociliary junction and are rarely visualized, even with wide dilation, only to be revealed with UBM imaging. Mid-zonal IPE cysts can appear as brown and fusiform with a dome-shaped appearance on the back of the iris. After dilation, the cyst may evert over the pupillary margin edge onto the iris stroma. Like neuroepithelial cysts, these tumors may be referred due to an asymptomatic iris stromal bulge with or without focal angle closure. Like all tumors located posterior to the iris, IPE cysts are best visualized by UBM or AS-OCT, which reveal their cystic internal characteristic. A small subset of dislodged IPE cysts are the rarest. They are either free-floating or, typically, stuck into the inferior anterior chamber angle, or in the vitreous and require no treatment. However, large IPE cyst–induced ACG must be treated with laser cystotomy. Nd:YAG (neodymium-doped yttrium aluminum garnet) laser cystotomy will deflate the cyst, releasing serous fluid.[29,30] It is important to rule out melanoma, including cyst and IPE adenoma, with each of these types of IPE prior to laser.[31]
- Iris stromal cysts can be congenital or acquired. They tend to have a characteristic clinical appearance with a smooth surface and a lucent mass on or within the stroma occasionally with fluid-debris level.[32] These tumors can be epithelial inclusion cyst, increase in size and spontaneously rupture causing secondary iritis, photophobia, pain, and glaucoma.[32]

Secondary iris cysts include epithelial (eg, postoperative, following trauma, epithelial downgrowth), pearl cyst, drug induced, or parasitic cysts. They can also be present secondary to solid intraocular tumors, like uveal melanoma or medulloepithelioma.[33]

Melanocytic Iris Tumors

Melanocytic tumors include freckle, nevus, melanocytoma, Lisch nodule, inflammatory nodules, and melanoma.[34]

- Freckle can be single or multifocal and usually rests on the iris stromal surface as a pigmented or nonpigmented lesion, typically 1 to 2 mm in diameter.[34]
- Nevus presents as focal areas of pigmentation that are either flat or minimally elevated. They may show comparatively deeper penetration in the iris stroma that causes dysmorphic

distortion. When iris nevi present with infiltration, iris distortion, corectopia, ectropion uveae, or sector cataract, they must be differentiated from iris melanomas.[34] UBM has been employed to help measure and thereby follow suspicious iris nevi for evidence of growth.[12-15] Typically, they appear as low reflective surface plaques overlying a thickened iris stroma.[15]

- Melanocytoma is a dark brown to black dome-shaped mass with minimal or no ectropion, often with a granular "mound of black sand" appearance.[31] They may show minor seeding into the anterior chamber angle or onto the iris stroma. Typically, anterior segment melanocytomas are non-progressive, asymptomatic, and do not cause secondary complications.[35] However, they can grow, cavitate, and shed pigment.[33] They can simulate uveal melanoma causing hyphema, corectopia, or intractable glaucoma.[35,36] A suspected melanocytoma may be observed for growth. If growth is documented the diagnosis of melanoma should be considered.[1] Biopsy can be helpful to establish the diagnosis.[33,35,]
- Iris melanoma is malignant with a metastatic rate of up to 11%.[37,38] The least common subtype of uveal melanoma, it comprises only up to 3% of cases.[37,39] Like choroidal melanoma, the age of presentation is in sixth decade of life with no sex predilection. The majority of iris melanomas develop from a pre-existing iris nevus and within the iris stroma.[40] They frequently originate in the peripupillary iris, then followed by midzone, and less frequently in the iris periphery.[41,42] The inferior quadrants are most commonly affected followed by the temporal, nasal, and superior quadrants.[1] They most commonly present as a solitary, tapioca-colored, nodular tumor with intrinsic vascularity.[14,43] Clinical features of include tumor vascularization, ectropion uvea, pupillary distortion, pigment dispersion, sector cataract, and glaucoma.[40,43,44] High-frequency ultrasound imaging (UBM) typically reveals a nodular arising from the iris surface or medium to highly reflective thickening of iris stroma.[1,13,14] For smaller tumors, documented growth is the most important feature for diagnosis. Most eye cancer specialists will base management on tumor size. Small, suspicious iris nevi or possible melanomas are photographed and measured with ultrasound, then carefully followed up at 3 to 6 month intervals to monitor for growth.[1] We suggest high-quality slit-lamp and gonio-photographs together with high-frequency ultrasound measurements with cross-sectional images (transverse and longitudinal) used to measure maximum tumor thickness (height) as well as longitudinal and transverse width. The differential diagnosis of iris melanomas include iris nevi, cysts, leiomyoma, metastases, and juvenile xanthogranulomas.[1,57] Medium and larger sized melanomas are more easy to diagnose. Here, a clinical diagnosis is often adequate. However, it can be augmented by biopsy with histopathological features analysis.
- The management of iris melanoma has depended upon several clinical features, including tumor size, location or extent, tumor seeding, and presence of tumor-related glaucoma.[38,46] Treatment options include iridectomy, iridocyclectomy, plaque brachytherapy, proton beam radiotherapy, and enucleation.[47] In consideration of the relative risks and benefits of intraocular resection surgery (eg, hemorrhage, long-term mydriatic glare, retinal detachment, lens dislocation, infection, inflammation) vs extraocular plaque radiation therapy (late cataract), there has been a shift toward plaque irradiation.[48,49]
- Ring and diffuse iris melanoma are rare varieties of uveal melanomas.[50] They often present with unilateral glaucoma and/or heterochromia. Gonioscopy shows infiltration of anterior chamber angle structures. Transillumination can reveal ring ciliary body involvement. Other clinical features include presence of sentinel vessels, ectropion uveae, iris heterochromia, and cataract.[50] Patients presenting with unilateral glaucoma with iris heterochromia should undergo high-frequency UBM. In case of suspicion, transcorneal fine-needle aspiration biopsy or iridectomy biopsy should be performed. Ring melanomas have been described to have large basal dimensions and thus carry a poor systemic and ocular prognosis.[51]

Nonmelanocytic Iris Tumors

Nonmelanocytic tumors include choristoma; tumors of vascular, fibrous, neural, myogenic, epithelial, or xanthomatous/xanthogranulomatous origin; metastases lymphoid, leukemic and secondary lesions; and nonneoplastic simulators.[16]

- The most commonly encountered vascular tumors of the iris are capillary hemangioma, iris cavernous hemangioma, iris microhemangioma, iris arteriovenous malformation, iris varix, and microhemangiomatosis.[20,52]
- Solid epithelial tumors are IPE adenoma, medulloepithelioma , and IPE adenocarcinoma.[1]
- Metastatic iris tumors include primary tumors originating from breast, lung, prostate, skin, kidney, colon, and thyroid.[1,16] Metastatic iris tumors are usually unilateral and may present with secondary glaucoma.[16]
- Nonneoplastic lesions simulating iris tumors include iridocorneal endothelial syndrome, iris atrophy, foreign body, iris coloboma, and heterochromia.[31]

Benign Versus Malignant Iris Tumors

The categories of iris tumors described previously have both benign and malignant subtypes.

Management

The management options for iris tumors include observation, local resection, and radiotherapy. As in the past, enucleation is employed for eyes with very large, malignant tumors where conservative therapies are not possible and/or when secondary glaucomatous has led to a blind and painful eye.[1] However, with the advent of advanced techniques, such as eye-sparing radiotherapy, physicians and patients prefer eye- and vision-sparing alternative treatments.

Observation

Most small melanocytic iris tumors can be observed for growth.[1] Lesions selected for observation must be well documented with high-quality slit-lamp and gonioscopic photographs to capture the tumor surface characteristics. Tumor size, boundaries, and reflectivity can be documented using transillumination and UBM.[2,5,6] Biopsy or treatment should be considered when growth is documented or leads to complications such as iris neovascularization and secondary glaucoma.

Local Resection

- Iridectomy: Sector/partial iridectomy includes removal of the tumor and margin of normal appearing iris. Solitary and localized iris tumors, such as melanocytoma or small melanomas, can be managed by sector iridectomy. Common complications include glare, anterior chamber hyphema, cataract, and intraocular pressure changes.[48]
- Iridocyclectomy: This technique includes removal of iridociliary tumor via a scleral flap. The main indications include iridociliary and ciliary tumors that usually don't respond well to radiotherapy such as adenoma and adenocarcinoma.[1] Local resection invariably causes a dysmorphic, dystonic pupil or large optical opening with associated anisocoria, accommodative symptoms, and photophobia.

Brachytherapy

The most commonly used radionuclides for brachytherapy of iris tumors include iodine-125 (^{125}I), palladium-103 (^{103}Pd), and ruthenium-106 (^{106}Ru).[1,49] Brachytherapy consists of suturing the radioactive plaque to cover over the tumor's base and a tumor-free perimeter of 2 to 3 mm.[49] The device is typically left in place for 4 to 7 days while the tumor receives the prescribed dose of radiation. Plaque brachytherapy is the most commonly used eye- and vision-sparing modality for malignant iris tumors.[43,49] Complications observed after plaque radiation therapy depend on the plaque source, dose and dose rate.[53] They include keratopathy, cataracts, scleral necrosis, rubeosis iridis, neovascular glaucoma, radiation vasculopathy, and radiation neuropathy.[1,39,43,49]

Proton Beam Irradiation

Proton beam irradiation can be used to effectively control most iris melanomas with reasonable chance of eye and vision retention.[54] Compared to brachytherapy, charged-particle radiation therapy delivers more irradiation to most anterior segment and adnexal structures.[49,54] Compared to plaque brachytherapy, proton-beam patient suffer more severe dry eye, lash loss and neovascular glaucoma.

Enucleation

Enucleation remains the standard treatment for tumors too large to be managed by local resection or irradiation, eyes with intractable glaucoma, and tumors unresponsive to radiation.[1,6,16,34]

In summary, iris tumors can be diagnosed with careful clinical evaluation. High-frequency ultrasonography and biopsy improve the diagnostic ability of the clinician. The management options depend upon tumor type, location, size, local extension, growth patterns, and related complications.

Iris Cysts

Iris cysts are benign lesions arising from the iris tissue and seen clinically in cyst or elevated form. They can be primary (with no etiological cause) or secondary (with etiological cause).

Primary Iris Cysts

Primary iris cysts are divided into epithelial and stromal types, depending upon their tissue of origin and clinical characteristics. Epithelial cysts arise between the pigmented epithelial layers of the iris. They can be central, peripheral, and middle part of iris in relation to the pupil. Primary stromal cysts arise within the stroma and are not in straight connection with the posterior epithelium.[28,55] They arise from the ectopic surface epithelium that is trapped in the iris during embryologic development.

Secondary Iris Cysts

Secondary iris cysts often arise after ocular trauma or surgery.

Free-Floating Cysts

Free-floating cysts are usually dislodged pigment epithelial cysts.

Spectrum of Presentations

Recurrent Cyst in Child

A 3-year-old girl with decreased vision since birth was diagnosed with an iris cyst on examination under anesthesia. She had undergone cystotomy twice and was shown to have recurrence after each time. On UBM, the cyst measured about 5 × 6 mm. There was corneal adhesion and scar formation. The lens was seen to be cataractous and tilted due to mechanical pressure from the overlying iris cyst. The patient underwent cystectomy with lensectomy and en bloc iridectomy under general anesthesia (Figure 16-1). A glued intraocular lens (IOL) was implanted. The patient may need future keratoplasty if corneal decompensation sets in. The postoperative period showed mild corneal edema with a nicely centered glued IOL.

Iris Cyst Causing Intraocular Lens Tilt

A 60-year-old man presented with blurred vision for the 6 months. He had a history of cataract surgery performed 3 years ago. On examination, he had a huge iris cyst arising from the epithelium. There was endothelial encroachment and corneal edema was present (Figure 16-2). The cyst was pressing on the posterior chamber IOL causing IOL tilt as seen in optical coherence tomography. The patient underwent cystectomy under local anesthesia.

Iris Cyst Following Keratoplasty

An 18-year-old woman presented with a history of blurred vision. She had optical penetrating keratoplasty performed at the age of 10 years for keratoconus. On examination, her best corrected visual acuity was 20/30 in the right eye and 20/80 in the left eye. Her previous records showed that her best corrected visual acuity was 20/40 in the left eye about 6 months ago. There was an inferior iris cyst observed with graft corneal endothelial touch and mild corneal edema (Figure 16-3). Nd:YAG cystotomy was performed, and she was administered an oral steroid course for 2 weeks.

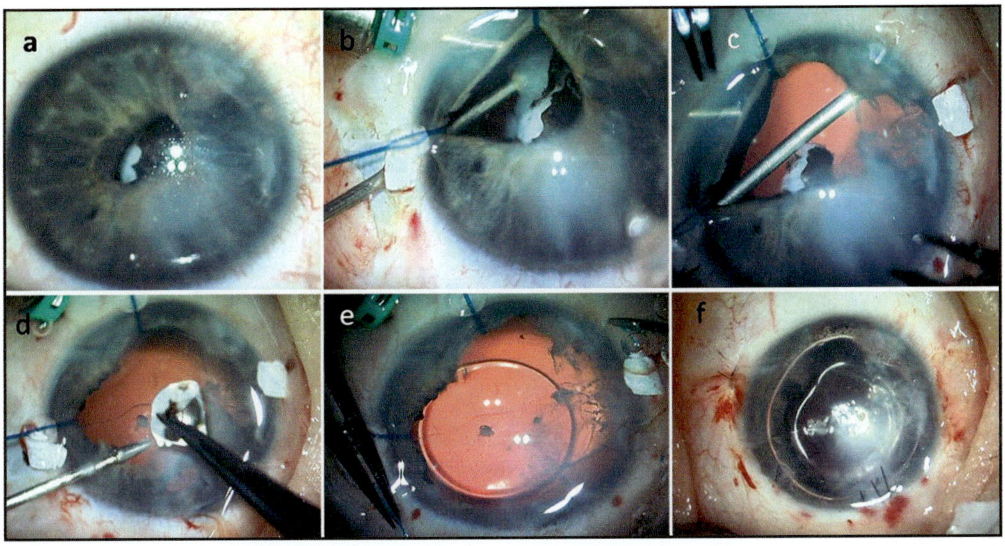

Figure 16-1. (A) Preoperative picture of the iris cyst. (B) Iris hooks placed and cystectomy performed with vitreous cutter. (C, D) Lensectomy, iridectomy, and cystectomy performed as en bloc excision. (E) Glued IOL implanted. (F) Air bubble injected and scleral flaps closed.

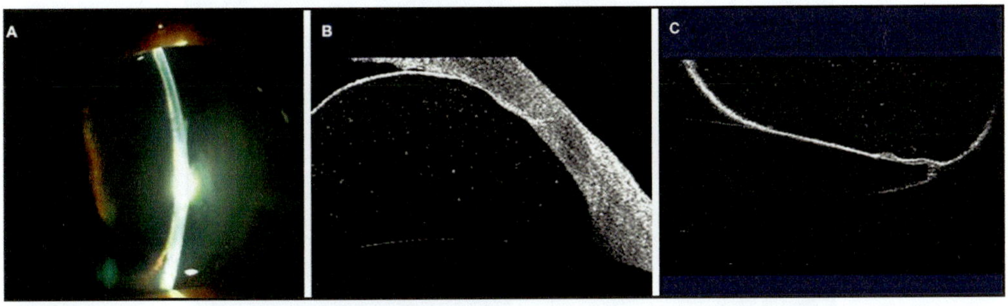

Figure 16-2. (A, B) Large serous iris cyst with corneal endothelial touch. (C) Cyst pressing on the IOL and inducing tilt.

Topical steroids and lubricants were continued for 1 month. Two months postoperatively, she showed clear cornea with best corrected visual acuity of 20/40.

Asymptomatic Iris Cyst

An iris cyst can be present in patients without any symptoms for a long period of time. Patients on routine examination for refractive or cataract surgery have been observed to have asymptomatic cysts (Figure 16-4). However, such iris cysts need not be intervened. Iris cyst can be large and present in a horseshoe shape (Figure 16-5). The large kissing cysts can, at times, induce a pinhole effect. Iris cysts arising from posterior pigment epithelium can mimic melanoma.

Diagnosis and Complications

Clinically, an iris cyst can be well observed on slit lamp; however, diagnostic information can be obtained by using imaging modalities like UBM or AS-OCT.[56] For example, UBM shows thick walls that are hyperechoic (eg, due to pigmented epithelium) or hypoechoic (eg, due to fluid content). UBM is superior to optical coherence tomography in such cases because the infrared light of the optical coherence tomography cannot pass through the iris pigment epithelium. In their initial phase, iris cysts can be silent, and later can induce iridocyclitis and ACG.[57] Chronic iris cysts induce endothelial decompensation due to corneal touch and cause corneal opacification. In cases

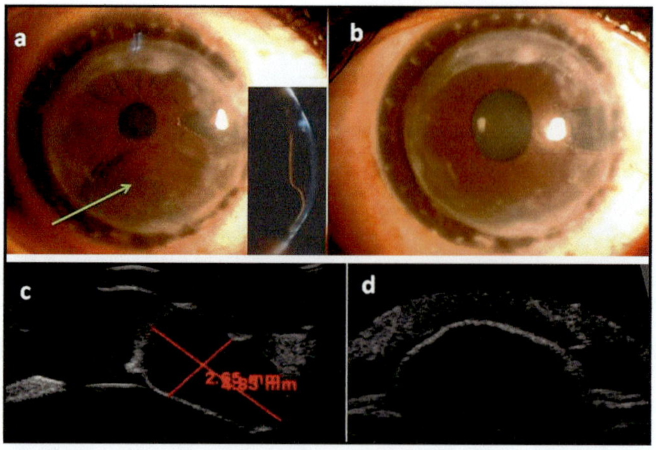

Figure 16-3. (A) Iris cyst and corneal edema following penetrating keratoplasty. (B) Postoperative Nd:YAG cystotomy. (C, D) UBM showing the cyst in situ and corneal graft touch.

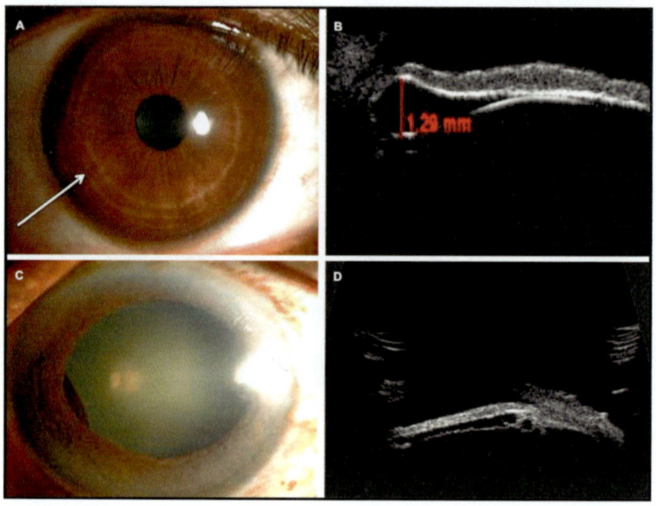

Figure 16-4. Asymptomatic iris cyst picture and UBM (A, B) in a patient undergoing LASIK workup and (C, D) a patient undergoing cataract workup.

of suspicious lesions, MRI may be advised. Early diagnosis and observation in asymptomatic cases may help; however, when vision-threatening complications are present, surgical removal or laser cystotomy is recommended.[58]

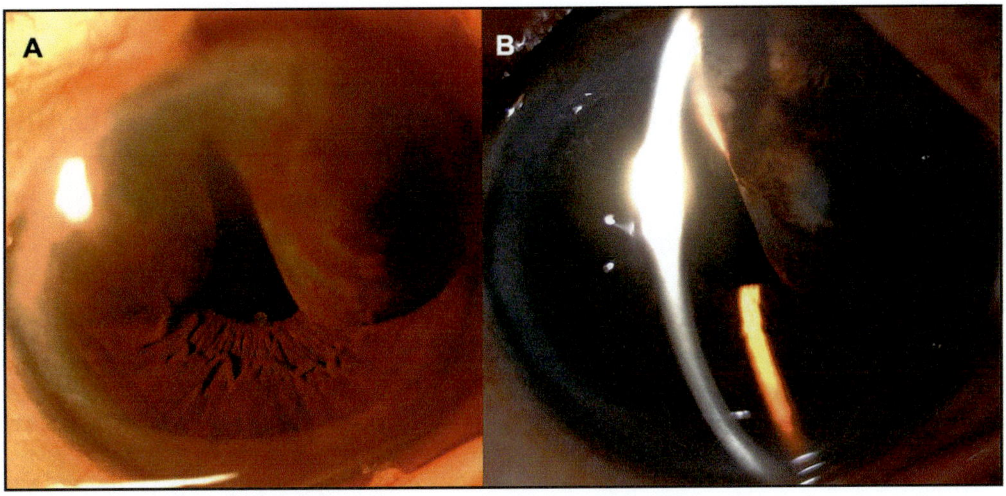

Figure 16-5. Asymptomatic large horseshoe iris cyst causing a pinhole effect.

Acknowledgment

Paul T. Finger, MD would like to thank The Eye Cancer Foundation for their support of all of his nonclinical work and worldwide fellowship program.

Case Presentation

Iris Pigment Epithelial Cyst Removal and Defect Repair

Dhivya Ashok Kumar, MD, FRCS, FICO, FAICO

A case of an IPE cyst that underwent cyst excision. This was followed by iris reconstruction and glued IOL implantation as the eye was aphakic with deficient capsules.

Under peribulbar anesthesia and sterile precaution, transscleral trocar cannula infusion was placed via pars plana about 3 mm from the limbus. Two conjunctival peritomies 180 degrees apart were performed at 11 and 5 clock hours (Figure 16-6A and Video 16-2). Subsequently, partial scleral flaps were made in lamellar fashion at 11 and 5 o'clock diagonally. Sclerotomy was made below the scleral flaps using a 22-gauge needle. A superior corneal incision was made via a 1.3-mm keratome. A rod was passed through the superior incision to retract the iris and visualize the underlying epithelial cyst and simultaneously a 23-gauge vitrector was passed through the sclerotomy opposite the cyst. The vitreous near the port, pupillary plane, and surrounding the cyst was cut initially. Then, under direct visualization, the cyst was excised by the vitrector (Figure 16-6B). Once the entire epithelium was removed anteriorly, a vitrectomy was performed in the pupillary plane and anterior chamber. A 3-piece foldable IOL was then implanted using the glued IOL method after extending the main incision via an injector. The leading haptic was introduced into the anterior chamber while a second instrument or glued IOL forceps was introduced through the sclerotomy site and the leading haptic grabbed and externalized beneath the scleral flaps using the handshake technique (Figure 16-6C). The trailing haptic was also externalized in a similar way under the scleral flaps. When both haptics were externalized, the haptics were tucked in the Scharioth tunnel at the point of externalization using 26-gauge needles.

Once the IOL was in place, the iris defect was sutured using a single-pass four-throw pupilloplasty (Figure 16-6D). Using the side port keratome, 2 stab incisions were made on either side of the limbus along the defect of the iris. The proximal iris defect was grasped with end-opening forceps (see Figure 16-6D) and the needle of the polypropylene single -armed suture passed. The distal end of the iris defect was grasped with end-opening forceps and the 26-gauge needle passed through it and railroaded through the needle. The Prolene (Ethicon) needle end was anchored onto the barrel of the needle on the opposite end and brought outside the eye. A Sinskey hook was then introduced inside the anterior chamber and a loop formed by hooking along the suture and the hook pulled through the opposite paracentesis. The suture end was then passed 4 times into the loop and the 2 ends pulled to approximate the knot that slides onto the iris in the anterior chamber. The suture ends were then cut within the anterior chamber. After the iris repair was completed, the scleral flaps were apposed using fibrin glue.

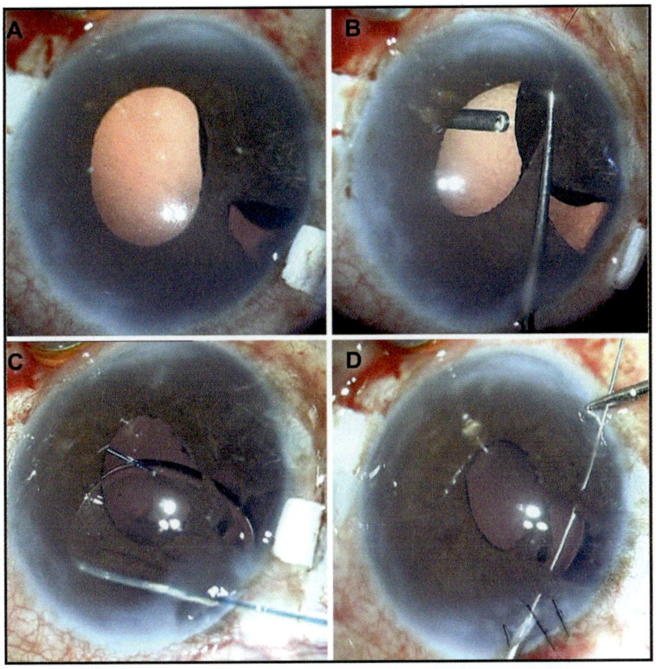

Figure 16-6. IPE cyst excision and iris repair with glued IOL. (A) Two scleral flaps made and infusion positioned. (B) After initial vitrectomy near the cyst and the port, the iris cyst is excised using the vitrector. (C) Glued transscleral fixated IOL is implanted. (D) Iris defect repaired by single-pass four-throw pupilloplasty.

References

1. Marigo FA, Finger PT. Anterior segment tumors: current concepts and innovations. *Surv Ophthalmol.* 2003;48(6):569-953.
2. Augsburger JJ, Affel LL, Benarosh DA. Ultrasound biomicroscopy of cystic lesions of the iris and ciliary body. *Trans Am Ophthalmol Soc.* 1996;94:259-274.
3. Iezzi R, Rosen RB, Tello C, et al. Personal computer-based 3-dimensional ultrasound biomicroscopy of the anterior segment. *Arch Ophthalmol.* 1996;114:520-524.
4. Marigo FA, Esaki K, Finger PT. Differential diagnosis of anterior segment cysts by ultrasound biomicroscopy. *Ophthalmology.* 1999;106:2131-2135.
5. Marigo FA, Finger PT, McCormick SA. Iris and ciliary body melanomas: ultrasound biomicroscopy with histopathologic correlation. *Arch Ophthalmol.* 2000;118:1515-1521.
6. Finger PT, Reddy S, Chin K. High-frequency ultrasound characteristics of 24 iris and iridociliary melanomas: before and after plaque brachytherapy. *Arch Ophthalmol.* 2007;125(8):1051-1058.
7. Bianciotto C, Shields CL, Guzman JM, Romanelli-Gobbi M, Mazzuca Jr D, Green WR, Shields JA. Assessment of anterior segment tumors with ultrasound biomicroscopy versus anterior segment optical coherence tomography in 200 cases. *Ophthalmology.* 2011;118(7):1297-1302.
8. Pavlin CJ, Vásquez LM, Lee R, et al. Anterior segment optical coherence tomography and ultrasound biomicroscopy in the imaging of anterior segment tumors. *Am J Ophthalmol.* 2009;147:214-219.
9. Siahmed K, Berges O, Desjardins L, et al. Anterior segment tumor imaging: advantages of ultrasound (10, 20 and 50 MHz) and optical coherence tomography. Article in French. *J Fr Ophtalmol.* 2004;27:169-173.
10. Augsburger JJ, Shields JA. Fine needle aspiration biopsy of solid intraocular tumors: indications, instrumentation and techniques. *Ophthalmic Surg.* 1984;15:34-40.
11. Finger PT, Latkany P, Kurli M, Iacob C. The Finger iridectomy technique: small incision biopsy of anterior segment tumors. *Br J Ophthalmol.* 2005;89(8):946-949.
12. Finger PT, McCormick SA, Lombardo J, et al. Epithelial inclusion cyst of the iris. *Arch Ophthalmol.* 1995;113:777-780.
13. Marigo FA, Esaki K, Finger PT. Differential diagnosis of anterior segment cysts by ultrasound biomicroscopy. *Ophthalmology.* 1999;106:2131-2135.
14. Marigo FA, Finger PT, McCormick SA. Iris and ciliary body melanomas: ultrasound biomicroscopy with histopathologic correlation. *Arch Ophthalmol.* 2000;118:1515-1521.
15. Marigo FA, Finger PT, McCormick SA. Anterior segment implantation cysts: ultrasound biomicroscopy with histopathologic correlation. *Arch Ophthalmol.* 1998;116:1569-1575.
16. Shields CL, Shields PW, Manalac J, Jumroendararasame C, Shields JA. Review of cystic and solid tumors of the iris. *Oman J Ophthalmol.* 2013;6(3):159.
17. Bandello F, Brancato R, Lattanzio R, et al. Biomicroscopy and fluorescein angiography of pigmented iris tumors: a retrospective study on 44 cases. *Int Ophthalmol.* 1994;18:61-70.
18. Brancato R, Bandello F, Lattanzio R. Iris fluorescein angiography in clinical practice. *Surv Ophthalmol.* 1997;42:41-70.
19. Dart JK, Marsh RJ, Garner A, Cooling RJ. Fluorescein angiography of anterior uveal melanocytic tumors. *Br J Ophthalmol.* 1988;72:326-337.
20. Jain P, Finger PT. Iris varix: 10-year experience with 28 eyes. *Indian J Ophthalmol.* 2019;67(3):350.
21. Price MJ, Bell RA, Willis WE, Whiteman DW. Tapioca melanoma of the iris: clinicopathological correlation with results of fluorescein angiography. *Can J Ophthalmol.* 1981;16:195-199.
22. Adam G, Brab M, Bohndorf K, Gunther RW. Gadolinium DTPA-enhanced MRI of intraocular tumors. *Magn Reson Imaging.* 1990;8:683-689.
23. Haik BG, Saint Louis L, Smith ME, et al. Magnetic resonance imaging in choroidal tumors. *Ann Ophthalmol.* 1987;19(6):218-222, 238.
24. Kuo MD, Hayman LA, Lee AG, et al. In vivo CT and MR appearance of prosthetic intraocular lens. *AJNR Am J Neuroradiol.* 1998;19(4):749-753.
25. Nakazawa T, Abe T, Sato Y, et al. Magnetic resonance imaging of a non-pigmented adenoma of the ciliary epithelium. *Acta Ophthalmol Scand.* 2000;78:470-473.
26. Grossniklaus HE. Fine-needle aspiration biopsy of the iris. *Arch Ophthalmol.* 1992;110:969-976.
27. Shields JA. Primary cysts of the iris. *Trans Am Ophthalmol Soc.* 1981;79:771-809.
28. Lois N, Shields CL, Shields JA, Mercado G. Primary cysts of the iris pigment epithelium: clinical features and natural course in 234 patients. *Ophthalmology.* 1998;105:1879-1885.
29. Kathil P, Chin KJ, Ghaznawi N, Finger PT. Transpupillary Nd: YAG laser cystotomy for iris pigment epithelial cysts with secondary progressive angle closure. *Ophthalmic Surg Lasers Imaging Retina.* 2011 Mar 24;42 Online:e40-43.
30. Xiao Y, Wang Y, Niu G, Li K. Transpupillary argon laser photocoagulation and Nd: YAG laser cystotomy for peripheral iris pigment epithelium cyst. *Am J Ophthalmol.* 2006;142(4):691-693.
31. Philip SS, John DR, Ninan F, John SS. Surgical management of post-traumatic iris cyst. *Open Ophthalmol J.* 2015;9:164-6.
32. Lois N, Shields CL, Shields JA, Mercado G. Primary iris stromal cysts: a report of 17 cases. *Ophthalmology.* 1998;105:1317-1322.
33. Kathil P, Milman T, Finger PT. Characteristics of anterior uveal melanocytomas in 17 cases. *Ophthalmology.* 2011;118(9):1874-1880.

34. Harbour JW, Augsburger JJ, Eagle RC Jr. Initial management and follow-up of melanocytic iris tumors. *Ophthalmology.* 1995;102:1987-1993.
35. Khadem JJ, Weiter JJ. Melanocytomas of the optic nerve and uvea. *Int Ophthalmol Clin.* 1997;37:149-158.
36. Biswas J, D'Souza C, Shanmugam MP. Diffuse melanotic lesion of the iris as a presenting feature of ciliary body melanocytoma: report of a case and review of the literature. *Surv Ophthalmol.* 1998;42:378-382.
37. Jensen OA. Malignant melanomas of the human uvea. Recent follow-up of cases in Denmark, 1943–1952. *Acta Ophthalmol* (Copenh). 1970;48(6):1113-1128.
38. Khan S, Finger PT, Yu GP et al. Clinical and pathologic characteristics of biopsy-proven iris melanoma: a multicenter international study. *Arch Ophthalmol.* 2012;130(1);57-64.
39. Shields CL, Shields JA, Materin M, Gershenbaum E, Singh AD, Smith A. Iris melanoma: risk factors for metastasis in 169 consecutive patients. *Ophthalmology.* 2001;108:172-178.
40. Kanski JJ. Tumors of the eye. In: *Clinical Ophthalmology: A Systematic Approach.* Oxford, United Kingdom: Butterworth-Heinemann; 1994:207.
41. Geisse LJ, Robertson DM. Iris melanomas. *Am J Ophthalmol.* 1985;99:638-648.
42. van Klink F, de Keizer RJ, Jager MJ, Kakebeeke-Kemme HM. Iris nevi and melanomas: a clinical follow-up study. *Doc Ophthalmol.* 1992;82:49-55.
43. Harbour JW, Augsburger JJ, Eagle RC Jr. Initial management and follow-up of melanocytic iris tumors. *Ophthalmology.* 1995;102:1987-1993.
44. Workman DM, Weiner JW. Melanocytic lesions of the iris—a clinocopathological study of 100 cases. *Aust N Z J Ophthalmol.* 1990;18:381-384.
45. Tomar AS, Finger PT, Iacob C. Intraocular leiomyoma: Current concepts. *Surv Ophtalmol.* 2020;65(4):421-437.
46. Shields JA, Sanborn GE, Ausburger JJ. The differential diagnosis of malignant melanoma of the iris. *Ophthalmology.* 1983;90:716-720.
47. Chaugule SS, Finger PT. Regression patterns of iris melanoma after Palladium-103 (^{103}Pd) plaque brachytherapy. *Ophthalmology.* 2017;124(7):1023-1030.
48. Conway RM, Chua WC, Qureshi C, Billson FA. Primary iris melanoma: diagnostic features and outcome of conservative surgical treatment. *Br J Ophthalmol.* 2001;85:848-854.
49. Finger PT. Plaque radiation therapy for malignant melanoma of the iris and ciliary body. *Am J Ophthalmol.* 2001;132:328-335.
50. Demirci H, Shields CL, Shields JA, et al. Ring melanoma of the anterior chamber angle: a report of fourteen cases. *Am J Ophthalmol.* 2001;132:336-342.
51. Shields CL, Di Nicola M, Bekerman VP, Kaliki S, Alarcon C, Fulco E, Shields JA. Iris melanoma outcomes based on the American Joint Committee on Cancer Classification in 432 patients. *Ophthalmology.* 2018;125(6):913-923.
52. Shields JA, Bianciotto CG, Kligman B, Shields CL. Vascular tumors of the iris: a review of 45 patients. The 2009 Helen Keller Lecture. *Arch Ophthalmol.* 2010;128:1107-1112.
53. Yousef YA, Finger PT. Lack of radiation maculopathy after palladium-103 plaque radiotherapy for iris melanoma. *Int J Radiat Oncol Biol Phys.* 2012;83(4):1107-1112. doi: 10.1016/j.ijrobp.2011.09.033
54. Gragoudas ES, Goitein M, Koehler A. Proton irradiation of malignant melanoma of the ciliary body. *Br J Ophthalmol.* 1979;63:135-139.
55. Gupta A, Pandian DG, Babu KR, Srinivasan R. Primary stromal iris cysts treated successfully with ab externo laser Nd:YAG photocoagulation. J Pediatr Ophthalmol Strabismus. 2010 Aug 23;47 Online:e1-4.
56. Pong JC, Lai JS. Imaging of primary cyst of the iris pigment epithelium using anterior segment OCT and ultrasonic biomicroscopy. Clin Exp Optom. 2009;92(2):139-141.
57. Tanihara H, Akita J, Honjo M, Honda Y. Angle closure caused by multiple, bilateral iridociliary cysts. *Acta Ophthalmol Scand.* 1997;75(2):216-217.
58. Kuchenbecker J, Motschmann M, Schmitz K, Behrens-Baumann W. Laser iridocystotomy for bilateral acute angle-closure glaucoma secondary to iris cysts. *Am J Ophthalmol.* 2000;129(3):391-393.

Please visit www.routledge.com/9781630917265

to access additional material.

Financial Disclosures

Dr. Amar Agarwal has no financial or proprietary interest in the materials presented herein.
Dr. Ashar Agarwal has no financial or proprietary interest in the materials presented herein.
Dr. Ashvin Agarwal has no financial or proprietary interest in the materials presented herein.
Dr. Athiya Agarwal has no financial or proprietary interest in the materials presented herein.
Dr. Masayuki Akimoto has no financial or proprietary interest in the materials presented herein.
Dr. Brandon D. Ayres has no financial or proprietary interest in the materials presented herein.
Dr. Sonal S. Chaugule has no financial or proprietary interest in the materials presented herein.
Dr. Robert J. Cionni has no financial or proprietary interest in the materials presented herein.
Dr. Alan S. Crandall has no financial or proprietary interest in the materials presented herein.
Dr. Paul T. Finger has no financial or proprietary interest in the materials presented herein.
Dr. Sadeer B. Hannush has no financial or proprietary interest in the materials presented herein.
Dr. Richard S. Hoffman has no financial or proprietary interest in the materials presented herein.
Dr. Santosh G. Honavar has no financial or proprietary interest in the materials presented herein
Dr. Dhivya Ashok Kumar has no financial or proprietary interest in the materials presented herein.
Dr. Ravi Kumar K V has no financial or proprietary interest in the materials presented herein.
Dr. Mami Kusaka has no financial or proprietary interest in the materials presented herein.
Dr. Yuri McKee has no financial or proprietary interest in the materials presented herein.
Dr. Kevin M. Miller has no financial or proprietary interest in the materials presented herein.
Dr. Priya Narang has no financial or proprietary interest in the materials presented herein.
Dr. Vladimir Pfeifer has no financial or proprietary interest in the materials presented herein.
Dr. Steven G. Safran has no financial or proprietary interest in the materials presented herein.
Dr. Michael E. Snyder is a consultant for and receives royalties from HumanOptics AG and is a shareholder in VEO Ophthalmics.

Dr. William B. Trattler has no financial or proprietary interest in the materials presented herein.

Dr. Claudio Trindade has a licence agreement with Morcher GmbH.

Dr. David T. Truong has no financial or proprietary interest in the materials presented herein.

Dr. Shin Yamane has no financial or proprietary interest in the materials presented herein.

Index

For Product Safety Concerns and Information please contact our
EU representative GPSR@taylorandfrancis.com Taylor & Francis
Verlag GmbH, Kaufingerstraße 24, 80331 München, Germany